LIVE FIT & FREE FOR LIFE: EXERCISE FOR SENIORS 60+

TARGETED EXERCISES THAT WILL INCREASE ENERGY, IMPROVE BALANCE, MOBILITY, AND STRENGTH IN 21 DAYS OR LESS

DR. ANDREA BLAKE-GARRETT

CONTENTS

INTRODUCTION

> "Aging is a fact of life. Looking your age doesn't have to be."
>
> — ANONYMOUS

Welcome to the journey of physical fitness and well-being! Your purchase of this book means that you self-identify as a senior. Congratulations! You have prioritized your health and wellness, especially in the years ahead. This book is your guide to unlocking the power of exercise and movement. Achieving physical fitness isn't just about looking good. It's about feeling great and maximizing the quality of your life. Research has shown that regular exercise can help reduce the effects of aging and can even avoid other age-related ailments. You'll learn more about how you can fight the effects of aging and illness as you read through the contents of this book. Ultimately, the goal of this book is to keep you moving. To help you remain healthy and active even as you age. Think Healthy!

You may not know this, but physical inactivity is one of the leading factors in people who experience obesity and chronic diseases. According to the World Health Organization (WHO), 23% of all adult deaths are caused by physical inactivity. It is estimated that 68% of all non-communicable diseases—a leading cause of death—could be prevented if physical activity was maintained. Obese individuals are especially vulnerable to cardiovascular disease, type 2 diabetes, and some cancers (WHO, 2018). Inactivity is also a risk factor for muscle and joint disorders due to a lack of physical exercise. Furthermore, inactive people are likely at higher risk for depression, anxiety, and increased stress (Biddle, Liu, Batterham, & Sallis, 2014). Additionally, physical inactivity has been associated with reduced cognitive function, which impairs problem-solving abilities (Alzheimer's Association, 2020).

Living longer and stronger is a common goal we both share. We can live longer by staying active and healthy as we age. Exercise is one of the best ways to maintain physical and mental well-being. Physical activity keeps our bodies strong and func-tioning and helps us maintain a positive mental attitude. Through exercise, we can improve our overall health, increase flexibility, decrease our risk for heart disease, reduce pain, boost energy levels, maintain independence, and even improve our quality of life. There are many ways for us to stay active and healthy as we age. I will explore some in the chapters ahead. It's essential for you to consult with your medical provider before beginning any new physical activity or exercise routine.

While growing older has its own unique set of challenges, it is still possible for seniors to add tremendous value to their future through exercise and nutrition. By incorporating various practices such as strength training, aerobics, stretching, social activities, and healthy eating, you can maintain your physical and mental health, stay independent, and live life to the fullest. Additionally, there are many social activities out there that can help you stay connected and build relationships while staying active. Group hikes, sports teams, and senior-friendly exercise classes are all excellent activities that allow you to stay healthy and connected with others.

Strength training is an integral part of any physical activity routine for seniors, as it can help build muscle strength, reduce the risk of falls, and improve balance. Low-impact aerobics activities like walking, swimming, tai chi, and yoga are also excellent forms of exercise and can help improve respiratory and cardiovascular health. Stretching is another great option to improve flexibility and range of motion. For those who have a chronic condition, low-impact activities can still benefit health. There are also modified exercises for you to use.

With this book, you will embark on an exercise journey towards a healthier, more sustainable life. In it, you will learn about age-appropriate exercises tailored explicitly for seniors 60 and older — from flexibility routines to weight-bearing activities, from balance training to aerobic conditioning. You will also learn about exercise's psychological and emotional benefits and how to incorporate them into your lifestyle.

No matter your shape, this book can help you achieve your fitness and performance goals. You'll learn the best exercises to target your needs and those of your peers. Routines are provided in Chapter 1. They will allow you to prepare in advance and practice as you continue learning in the following chapters.

No longer are the days of being bound to an inactive lifestyle. You can now join the expanding community of active seniors who find joy in movement and improved quality of life. So don't delay—read Chapter 1 first. As you complete the 21-day routine, continue through the rest of this book. Increased mobility, balance, and strength can be part of your happy and healthy life today!

Other books on Exercise for Seniors are on the market; thank you for choosing this one. Every effort was made to ensure it contained useful and valuable information. Please use and enjoy it. Dominate your life!

1

AT-HOME EXERCISES

Age is no barrier. It's a limitation you put on your mind."

— JACKIE JOYNER KERSEE

As we age, our bodies undergo many physical changes that can affect our overall health and mobility. That's why it's so important for seniors to stay active and engage in moving as many muscles as possible as they grow older. In this chapter, I will discuss sample workout and stretching routines designed with you in mind and some tips to help you stay motivated and get the most out of your workout routines. Also, these workouts and stretches will allow you to perform within the comforts of where you live. They can be completed using your body's weight. There's no need to visit fitness centers or use complicated gym equipment. You can use weights if you are able. As your strength increase, increase your weights. I purposefully designed these workouts so you can work out three to six times weekly using these three routines. At the end of twenty-one days of regular daily exercise, you will already be able to feel and see the benefits of moving frequently and staying active. Include a healthier diet to maximize your results!

Finally, I will provide some advice on staying committed and motivated to your workout routine and offer tips for making the most out of it. Keep in mind that consistency is critical. Whether you are a beginner looking to get into shape, or an experienced fitness enthusiast looking to stay in shape as you age, this book will add value, serving as a resource to get the most out of your exercise routine. So let's get started!

WORKOUT ROUTINE 1

One exercise can make a difference! Try one or more to build your workout routine. Consult your doctor to determine if any of these exercises are inappropriate for you. If any prior health conditions or physical limitations must be considered, modify them.

Warm Ups

1. Start with 10 minutes of light cardio, such as walking or seated cycling.
2. Stretch all your major muscle groups to work on improving flexibility.

Safety Precaution: Consult your physician to determine if these exercises are appropriate given your health conditions or physical limitations.

Balance Drills

1. Stand on one leg and hold the position for 30 seconds to 1 minute. The key is to keep one leg off the floor. That leg could be slightly bent backward or extended forwards.
2. Do three sets of the balance drill.

Safety Precaution: Use the wall, a chair, or a table to help support you, if necessary. Increase the repetitions of the one-leg balance drill gradually to reduce the chances of strain or injury.

Squats

1. Stand with legs shoulder width apart and feet parallel.
2. Push your hips back, bend your knees, and lower down until your thighs parallel the ground as if sitting down. If you are not able to squat that low, do the best that you can.
3. Return to the starting position, squeezing your glutes as you stand.
4. Do 10 - 15 reps with a slow and controlled motion. That is one rep.

Safety Precaution:

1. Pay attention to your body.
2. Stop immediately if you experience any knee pain or discomfort. You can modify squats by using a chair.
3. In a slow and controlled manner, sit in the chair and stand up.

Lunges

1. Stand with feet shoulder-width apart and step one foot forward.
2. Lower your back knee until it almost touches the ground or as far as possible. Raise your arms above your head or place them on your hips for balance.
3. Push back using the front leg, return to the starting position, and do the other side.
4. Do ten reps on each side.

Safety Precaution: Use the wall, a chair, or a table to help support you, if necessary. Build up the repetitions of the one-leg balance drill gradually to reduce the chances of strain or injury.

Step-Ups

1. Find a raised surface, such as the bottom step of a staircase or stepper, and place one foot on it.
2. Drive off the heel of the standing foot to raise your body up, bringing the other foot up to the same level.

3. Return to the starting position, and repeat on the other side.
4. Do ten reps on each side.

Safety Precaution: Stop performing the exercise if dizziness, lightheadedness, or pain occurs.

Push-Ups

1. Lay down on the ground/floor, with your feet on the ground/floor and hands directly underneath your shoulders.
2. Push through your palms and extend your arms to raise your body.
3. Return to the starting position and do ten reps.

Safety Precaution: If you cannot perform a full push-up, you can do a wall push-up for modification. Eventually, with enough practice, you will gain strength. You gradually challenge yourself to work up to a full push-up off the floor.

Planks

1. Lay down on the ground and prop yourself up on your palms and toes for a straight-arm plank. A forearm plank requires you to lower to arms until the elbow palm area sits firmly on the ground. Be sure to breathe slow, controlled breaths.
2. Squeeze your abs and glutes and keep your body straight.

3. Hold this position for 30 seconds to 1 minute.
4. Perform three sets.

Safety Precaution:

1. Keep the stomach muscles contracted and the back straight as possible, and avoid arching the spine.
2. Take breaks as needed and rest in-between sets.
3. Use a bench, table, or wall as a modification.

WORKOUT ROUTINE 2

One exercise can make a difference! Try one or more to build your workout routine. Consult your doctor to determine if any of these exercises are inappropriate for you. If any prior health conditions or physical limitations must be considered, modify them.

Warm Up

1. Start with 2 minutes of jogging in place, 1 minute of jumping Jacks, one minute-high knee, and 1 minute butt kicks.
2. Stretch all your major muscle groups and work on improving flexibility.

Chair Squats

1. Start squats by sitting in a chair with your feet hip-width apart and arms by your side.
2. Engage your core and slowly stand up from the chair while squeezing your glutes.
3. Once you have stood upright, sit back down slowly in the chair.
4. Aim to do 12-15 reps of these.

Safety Precautions: Make sure your chair is sturdy and that you have a good grip on the arms of the chair to help you stand up. You don't need to stand completely up out of the chair; hover above the seat so your knees don't go past your toes.

Seated Torso Twists

1. Begin seated in a chair with feet flat on the floor.
2. Place your hands over your chest, keeping your core engaged.
3. Twist your torso to the left, hold for a count of 5, and slowly twist to the right.
4. Your head should be in the direction of the twist, in alignment with your upper body. Try to complete 10-12 repetitions. Left and right is one repetition.

Safety Precautions: You must keep your back in line with your torso as you twist your body. Be sure to take controlled breaths - in through the nose, out through the mouth.

Glute Bridge

1. Begin by lying on your back, with feet flat, legs bent at a 45-degree angle, and hip-width apart.
2. Raise your hips off the floor, engaging the core.
3. Squeeze your glutes and hold at the top for 3-5 seconds.
4. Slowly lower your body back down to the floor.
5. Try to complete ten repetitions.

Safety Precautions: Ensure your back stays aligned with your shoulders throughout the motion.

Wall Sit

1. Begin by standing up against a wall, foot flat and hip-width apart.
2. Slowly slide your back down the wall until your thighs parallel the floor or as far as possible.
3. Make sure your core is engaged throughout the exercise.
4. Hold the position for 10 seconds and slowly slide back to standing.
5. Try to complete ten repetitions.

Safety Precautions: Take it easy if feeling any discomfort; sit higher.

Seated Knee Extension

1. Begin seated in a chair with feet flat on the floor.
2. Slowly extend your legs before you while keeping your back straight and core engaged.
3. With the leg extended and lifted slightly off the chair, point your toes up, if possible.
4. Hold for 1-2 seconds and slowly lower your legs back down to the starting position.
5. Try to complete ten repetitions.

Safety Precautions: Make sure the chair or bench is sturdy and placed firmly on the floor. Do not rock your back side to side or behind the chair.

WORKOUT ROUTINE 3

One exercise can make a difference! Try one or more to build your workout routine. Consult your doctor to determine if any of these exercises are inappropriate for you. If any prior health conditions or physical limitations must be considered, modify them.

Warm Up

1. Start with 10 minutes of light cardio, such as walking or seated cycling.
2. Stretch all your major muscle groups and work on improving flexibility.

Seated Core Strength

1. Begin by sitting on the chair with feet hip-width apart. The knees and feet are pointing out straight.
2. Raise your arms straight above your head and hold for 30-60 seconds. Beginners shoot for 30 seconds. Advanced 1 minute is your goal.
3. After a 15-second rest. Repeat. This time includes alternating knee raises for 30 – 60 seconds.
4. After a 15-second rest, hold your arms straight out in front of your body seated position, back and upper body straight. Bend forward at the hip, hold for 1 second, and return. Squeeze your abs. Do not bend your back. Keep it straight.
5. Repeat this rocking motion 15 – 20 times.

Safety Precautions: Make sure the chair or bench is sturdy and placed firmly on the floor.

Seated Toe / Heel Lifts

1. Sit with your feet facing forward and hip-width apart.
2. Slowly lift the toes of your feet up toward you and hold for two seconds.
3. Slowly lower your toes and repeat 10-12 times.
4. Repeat in the other direction.
5. Slowly lift your heel up toward you and hold for two seconds.
6. Slowly lower your toes and repeat 10-12 times.

Safety Precaution: Make sure the chair or bench is sturdy and placed firmly on the floor.

Bridge with Leg Lifts

1. Start by lying on your back with your knees bent and feet flat on the ground.
2. Squeeze your glutes and lift your hips as high as possible.
3. Once your bridge is in place, lift one leg straight and lower it.
4. Alternate legs and aim to do ten reps on each side.

Safety Precautions: Modify this by doing a bridge without the straight leg lift until you become stronger. Ensure you have a secure surface and a good grip on the floor to prevent slipping.

Wall Push-Ups

1. Place your hands flat against a wall and stand arm's length away.
2. Keeping your back straight, bend your elbows and lower yourself toward the wall. The rest of your body remains in a straight line.
3. Hold this position and then push back to the starting position.
4. Aim to do 10-15 reps of these.

Safety Precaution: Ensure your wall is secure and your feet are placed firmly on the ground to prevent slipping and ensure a safe position.

Seated Alternating Arm and Leg Raise

1. Start by sitting in a chair with your feet hip-width apart and arms stretched in front of you.
2. Raise one arm and one leg off the ground (left leg, right arm or right leg, left arm) and hold for two seconds.
3. Slowly lower back down and alternate sides (left leg, right arm or right leg, left arm).
4. Aim to do ten reps on each side.

Safety Precaution: Make sure your chair is sturdy and has a secure grip for support.

STRETCHING

This exercise is a full-body stretching routine that you can do to cool yourself down after every workout.

Seated Hamstring Stretch

1. Sit with one leg straight out in front, toes pointed up.
2. Reach for your toes with your hands and lean forward, keeping your back straight.
3. You should feel a mild to moderate stretch in the backs of your legs.
4. Hold for 15-20 seconds and then switch sides.

Standing Shin Stretch

1. Stand up with feet slightly wider than hip-width apart.
2. Balance on one leg and extend the other leg, pointing your toes towards the ceiling.
3. Reach down and grab the top of your foot, ankle, or shin with the opposite hand. Do not pull back on your toes. Just hold.
4. Press your knee toward the ground until you feel a light stretch in the back of the leg, shin, and ankle.
5. Hold for 15-20 seconds and then switch sides.

Standing Calf Stretch

1. Stand with both feet hip-width apart and face a wall.
2. Place both palms against the wall and lean forward.
3. Bend your knees until you feel a mild stretch through the calf muscles.
4. Hold for 15-20 seconds and then release. Repeat twice.

Seated Spinal Twist

1. Sit in a comfortable cross-legged position.
2. Place your left hand on your right knee and rotate the trunk of your body to the right, attempting to keep your upper body and head straight in the direction of the twist.
3. Hold for 15-20 seconds and then switch sides.

Towel Neck Stretch

1. Sit comfortably on the floor, chair, or bench with a towel behind your head.
2. With both elbows squared, grab the ends of the towel with your hands.
3. Gently pull the towel back and down, feeling a light stretch across your shoulders and upper back.
4. Hold for 15-20 seconds and then release.

Seated Forward Bend

1. Sit on the floor with your legs extended in front of you.
2. Reach for your toes and keep your back straight and your neck relaxed.
3. Feel a light stretch at the back of your legs. Hold for 15-20 seconds and then release.

Standing Forward Bend

1. Stand up straight. Legs shoulder width apart.
2. Extend your arm straight out as you bend towards the ground.
3. Reach for your toes and keep your back straight and your neck relaxed.
4. You should feel a light stretch at the back of your legs. Remember to breathe. Hold for 15-20 seconds and then release.

Tips to Stay Motivated

Regular exercise can be challenging, especially if you lack the self-motivation to get you going and stay that way. Finding the time and energy for an exercise routine can seem impossible, but you can build a consistent workout routine when you know how to stay motivated. I am sure you have heard the saying, "Mindset matters." It is true. In my book "DOWN 100 POUNDS: How I Use Positive Affirmations To Transform My Mind & Help Maximize My Weight Loss," I share the process that helped me achieve and maintain the right mindset for my 100-pound weight loss journey. In this segment, I'll share tips that can help you stay motivated and get the most out of your workout. Whether you're a beginner or advanced, these suggestions can make all the difference when finding the motivation to get physical.

Find Simple Ways to Make Exercise Fun

Exercise isn't always seen as an enjoyable activity. You will have to put in the work to achieve the results you want. It is an essential part of a healthy lifestyle. All movement is good! Finding ways to make exercise fun can help you stick to a routine and get in the physical activity you need. You want to engage as many muscles as possible. Variety is the spice of life! Do you like to dance? Do that! Play your favorite music and have a party 3-5 times a week. The main objective is to be consistent.

Switch it up! Trying various activities keeps exercise exciting and can be more stimulating for the mind and body. You can try walking, tai chi, dance classes, swimming, or cycling. Gather some family and friends and form a team. Don't have one? Join my team on Instagram at Teamnoexcuses50 "Notorious DRABG." Everyone likes to be rewarded for doing a good job, so give yourself a little incentive to keep going. Celebrate your daily and weekly triumphs. A small reward each time you reach a particular goal can help you stay motivated and have fun at the same time. Be kind to yourself. Exercise doesn't have to be a chore. Incorporating these tips can make exercise more enjoyable and help you stay active and healthy.

Don't Find Time, Make Time

It would be best to prioritize exercise in your daily routine instead of trying to find time to fit it in. Treat it as a lover you must see every day. Even if you only have 10-20 minutes to spare, including some form of exercise in your day will pay off for overall health and well-being. If time is an issue, try breaking up a workout into small chunks, such as a 15-minute walk in the morning and evening. BAM! That's 30 minutes that day. Break up the routine so you can adjust each segment's length to fit your schedule and preferences. Remember that any purposeful movement counts, whether jogging, walking, biking, yoga, or swimming. Attempting to exercise every day, even if it's only for 10-15 minutes, will help seniors to stay in better physical shape and can make a big difference in how they feel. So, no more excuses: make time to work out and move your body today!

Turn Exercise Into a Social Activity

Try turning exercise into a social activity as much as possible to stick to a routine and reap the health benefits. Build your consistency. A great way to make exercise a social movement is by joining an exercise class or a fitness group. A group of like-minded people can help you stay engaged, inspired, motivated, and accountable. It can also be an excellent opportunity to make new friends and maintain relationships. If group exercise classes aren't for you, try walking with a friend simultaneously each day or joining a virtual group. Create a Facebook or Instagram page and invite people to follow or join you.

Keep Track of Your Progress

It would be best to actively keep track of your progress to stay motivated and focused on your exercise routine. This can be done by measuring one's performance or progress each time you exercise. Set your goals at the start of each fitness session, and note any changes in performance or fitness levels. This can provide you with an objective point of departure for future workouts and offer incentives for pushing yourself harder and increasing exercise intensity.

A word of caution. Stay off the scale. Measure your progress in non-scalable ways. Have a pair of pants or a dress that is too small. Take monthly pictures wearing the same clothes. Try it on each month. Take inventory of how your body feels. Are you getting stronger? Can you walk faster or for more extended periods? Do you see muscles forming? Is your body feeling less heavy? Celebrate every triumph!

CONCLUSION

The benefits of regular physical activity are many. For you, not only is it essential as a means of preventing injury but also as a way to promote overall well-being. The different workout routines outlined in this chapter and throughout this book will provide options to explore and experiment with. If you are willing to invest your time and energy into your physical fitness now, you will continue to live free and fit later. You are reaping the benefits of improved body strength, balance, flexibility, and mental well-being. Whether it's light stretching, a full-body workout, or gentle yoga, find an exercise and nutrition routine that works for you and stick to it. The consistent person is one who always wins.

2

BALANCE

Balance can become more precarious as we age, increasing the risk of falls and serious injury. Balance exercises are an effective way to reduce this risk and improve mobility and physical function. In this chapter, I'll discuss the importance of balance training for seniors, provide an overview of the most beneficial exercises, and show examples of specific exercises. In addition, I'll explain the proper safety protocols to follow when exercising to ensure that everyone can stay safe and healthy. I hope this chapter provides helpful tips and exercises to help seniors maintain and improve their balance.

Did you know that the inner ear plays a vital role in maintaining balance by housing the vestibular system? Disruptions to the vestibular system can cause blurred vision, dizziness, unsteadiness, and nausea, among other symptoms. This system consists of two structures: the semicircular canals and the otoliths. The semicircular canals are three looping structures within the skull's temporal bone that sense angular acceleration, like turning or tilting of the head. The otoliths are two structures that sense linear acceleration, like forwarding and backward head movements.

The inner ear's vestibular system communicates with the brain to provide a sense of balance. When the head moves in any direction, fluid within the semicircular canals and otoliths stimulates the sensory cells. The sensory cells then signal the brain, which interprets this signal, allowing the person to maintain balance. Without the inner ear, a person would be unable to judge the position of their body in space or maintain balance.

Aside from that, migraines are often linked with balance problems due to dizziness, lightheadedness, and vertigo. These symptoms can disrupt the body's sense of balance by interfering with the vestibular system, which is responsible for our sense of equilibrium. When this system is affected, it can lead to disorientation, instability, and a spinning sensation. In addition, some studies have shown that migraineurs may have a heightened sensitivity to balance stimuli, making it more challenging to maintain equilibrium. Furthermore, certain medications used to treat migraines can lead to increased balance problems. Therefore, people with migraines should be aware of any balance issues they are experiencing and speak to their doctor about any concerns.

Fortunately, there is a way for you to continually work on your balance to improve your quality of life. The muscles, joints, and skin all work together to help the body maintain balance.

Muscles allow the body to make quick movements to balance itself. Joints are the connection points between bones, allowing the body to twist, turn, and bend to maintain balance. The skin helps provide sensory feedback to the brain, which enables the brain to assess the body's position and adjust accordingly to maintain balance. In addition, the inner ear's various structures help provide information about the body's function. They play an important role in helping your body to balance itself. All these components work together to help your body stay upright and balanced.

THE HUMAN BALANCE SYSTEM

The human balance system is an amazingly complex network of body parts that help us maintain equilibrium—consisting of multiple sensory and motor control systems, most notably the proprioceptive, vestibular, and visual systems. In this segment of the chapter, I will explore how these systems come together to allow us to maintain balance.

What Is Balance?

Balance is the ability to maintain equilibrium and coordination in the body and to respond quickly and effectively to any changes in the body's position or orientation. It is crucial for daily functioning because it helps you move more safely, stay upright, and maintain stability in various environments. By having good balance, you can make smoother movements, perform activities with greater accuracy and coordination, and prevent falls.

In the human balance system, balance is the ability to maintain an upright posture and the body's center of gravity over the base of support (feet). The human balance system comprises vestibular, proprioceptive, and visual components. The vestibular system detects head and body movements, while the proprioceptive system detects the body's orientation in space and muscle tension. The visual system acts as a check and provides information regarding the external environment. When these three systems work together correctly, they allow our body to stay balanced and upright.

Sensory Input

The muscle and joint input contributes to the human balance system by providing sensory information. The muscles, tendons, and joints work together to send signals to the brain that give information on the body's movements and position. The brain then adjusts the body's posture to maintain balance. With this information, the brain can adjust the tension of the muscles to respond to changes in the environment and to remain upright.

The vestibular system also helps to maintain human balance by providing information about head orientation, angular and linear acceleration, and deceleration to the brain and the central nervous system. This information is then used to determine the positioning of the head and neck in relation to gravity and to adjust the body's position accordingly. The vestibular system also sends messages to the muscles of the eyes, which assists in gaze stability and visual tracking.

Integrating sensory input into the human balance system involves coordinating multiple sensory systems. Visual input helps the body maintain balance by providing information on the location of objects in space. While another system helps detect movement and acceleration, another provides information on foot placement and muscle tension. A sensory system contributes to the awareness of body position and movement. All these senses work together to provide feedback to the brain, allowing your body to regulate balanced responses.

Unfortunately, there will be times wherein certain senses and signals will be misinterpreted by the body and result in balance conflict causing internal confusion and instability. To maintain balance, the brain constantly compares visual, auditory, and proprioceptive information to keep equilibrium. The processing of conflicting sensory information causes the brain finds it difficult to process the data and maintain balance. As a result, some may experience dizziness, vertigo, and nausea. In extreme cases, an individual may faint as the signals become too confusing for the brain, and the body's autonomic response systems struggle to keep up.

Motor Output

Motor output to the muscles, joints, and eyes results from a complex process of information gathered by the body's balance system. This process involves collecting sensory information from muscles, joints, and eyes and centralizing the data to determine how best to move the body. The balance system then uses this information to generate and direct muscular activity to produce an appropriate movement to maintain balance and stability.

Muscles contract and relax when the body senses an imbalance to provide a corrective force. For example, when the body leans forward, the balance system cause muscles in the back, abdominals, and hamstrings to contract. This causes the body to lean back and restore its balance. Regarding eye movement, the eyes help the body maintain its balance. When the body leans forward, the eyes focus on the ground in front and provide feedback to the balance system allowing it to maintain balance. The joint movement helps to sense and adjust body angles to provide a stable base.

The reception of all these sensory information results in motor output which is the activation of the muscles, joint movements, and eye movements that make up the body's movement, which, when coordinated, helps keep the body stable. This output is essentially an output of decisions made by the balance system to move the body in the right direction or to resist a disturbance in the right direction. As the body's sensory data changes, so does the motor output of its muscles, joints, and eyes.

WHY YOUR BALANCE WORSENS WITH AGE

Age-related changes to our bodies affect everything. Our reflexes, coordination, and muscle strength can weaken, and our joints can become stiffer and less flexible, making it more challenging to keep our balance. Some experience a natural progressive decline in physical and cognitive abilities. Sensory information used to maintain balance can be affected by body changes. For example, vision can be affected by cataracts or glaucoma, while hearing can be affected by age-related hearing loss.

Calcium deposits and degeneration of the hair cells that sense movement can affect the inner ear, leading to difficulty in spatially detecting the body's motion. It becomes difficult to determine where the body is with the ground. Age-related changes in the parts of the brain responsible for controlling balance, such as the cerebellum and the neurons in the brain stem and primary motor cortex, can also lead to worsened balance.

As you age, balance can inevitably decline, affecting your ability to move and perform everyday tasks.

All is not lost. There are a few simple yet effective ways to help improve and maintain your balance as you age. Exercise and physical activity can help increase muscle strength and coordination. Activities like step classes, yoga, tai chi, swimming, and a routine including heel and toe raises, one-leg stands, and squats are great for improving balance. Eating a healthy diet can help boost energy and improve balance. Ensure to include plenty of fruits and vegetables in your diet, as they are an excellent source of antioxidants. Getting enough sleep can also benefit your overall ability to maintain balance. Especially as we age, it's essential to take care of ourselves and make sure we are doing the best we can to keep our balance.

THE IMPORTANCE OF BALANCE TRAINING

Balance training is critical for everyone at any age, from young children to older people. For those who are younger and in their prime, balance training helps to increase focus and coordination. It also helps to improve stability and overall balance. Balance training can be beneficial when playing sports, as it can reduce the risk of injuries due to poor balance. Furthermore, balance training helps develop stronger muscles, improving overall coordination and agility.

For those who are older, balance training is even more critical, as it can reduce the risk of falls, which can result in serious injury. Balance training can help enhance the brain-body connection, which will help improve balance, posture, and coordination. Balance training can also help strengthen the muscles, improving overall stability.

Balance training is essential to any physical activity routine and is especially important for seniors. With age, the body's natural balance starts to deteriorate, and this can increase the risk of injury from falls. This type of training helps maintain and improve balance, coordination, and stability. It can also help to improve physical strength and flexibility.

Incorporating balance training into a routine can help prevent falls and avoid potentially serious injuries. An effective balance training program should include exercises that measure and improve posture, static and dynamic balance, and reaction time. Such activities can consist of standing on one leg, walking heel to toe, standing on an unstable surface, and doing exercises that involve moving an arm or leg. At the same time, the other side of the body remains stationary.

In addition to strength and balance exercises, proprioception or kinesthesia exercises can also be incorporated into your routine. Proprioception exercises involve specific movements or activities designed to improve the joint's ability to detect where it is in space. They reduce the risk of the joint moving beyond its range of motion which could lead to injury. Examples of proprioception exercises include single-leg balance exercises, lateral stepping exercises, and agility drills. Incorporating these exercises into your routine can help improve the strength and stability of your joints and reduce the risk of injury.

Balance training helps to improve one's ability to coordinate and control their body movement in space, which is an essential factor to consider when it comes to body awareness. As you age, you may become more unsteady on your feet, leading to falls. Balance training exercises can help improve your understanding of body position and movement in space, increase strength, coordination, and joint stability, and improve posture and body control.

IMPROVING YOUR BALANCE

As you age, it is natural for your balance to begin to deteriorate. But even though balance might deteriorate, you can still find ways to improve your equilibrium and avoid falls. With a little effort and dedication, it is possible to improve balance and prevent falls eliminating the risk of injury.

Step 1: Get Moving

To fight the harmful effects of aging, you should maintain a lifestyle that promotes healthy movement. Regular physical activity is essential for maintaining a healthy body and mind as we age. Staying active is vital to maintaining strength and mental acuity. It can also help to reduce joint pain and improve overall mobility. Doing light to moderate workouts three to four times weekly will help keep muscles strong and joints flexible.

If you choose not to live a very active lifestyle, other alternatives exist, such as yoga, stretching, gardening, and even light housework. It is beneficial to choose an enjoyable activity, as this will help motivate them to stay consistently active. When engaging in any action, you need to start slowly. Your physician or physical therapist should be consulted when starting any new exercise program. It is also important to gradually build intensity and duration while taking breaks when needed.

Finally, remember to stay safe when exercising. Wearing suitable clothing, using proper safety gear, stretching beforehand, taking 20-30 second breaks between exercises, and cooling down afterward can help prevent injuries.

Step 2: Do Specific Balance Exercises

Aside from generally staying active, you need to perform specific exercises to improve your balance as you age. Balance exercises help you improve your coordination and stability while sitting, standing, or walking. Examples include single-leg balancing, tandem standing, toe stands, and side steps. These exercises require you to work against the force of gravity, thereby strengthening the muscles responsible for keeping your balance. Additionally, these exercises help to stimulate the reflexes responsible for maintaining an upright posture and help to increase the individual's awareness of their body in space.

Strengthening exercises can also be useful as they can help you build the strength of the muscles used to maintain balance. Examples may include: squats, lunges, sit-to-stands, single-leg stands, and heel raises. These exercises help break the instability cycle of weak muscles, joints, and reflexes. Be sure to use your core and breathe deeply. As you age, it is essential for you to stay active and incorporate balance-improving exercises into your daily routine to stay safe and independent.

Step 3: Always Challenge Yourself

As we age, it's natural to want to slow down and enjoy the quiet pace of retirement. For many, however, this can be a mistake when not exercising regularly. Even as we age, we must challenge our bodies with various exercises that help keep us strong, flexible, and mobile.

You can help reduce the risk of age-related illnesses and boost cognitive abilities by challenging yourselves. Various physical activities, including strength training, stretching, balance and coordination exercises, and aerobic and anaerobic exercises, can help you stay fit and fine.

Strength training is a crucial component for maintaining muscle mass and bone density. Weight machines, resistance bands, or body weights can help build strength. For seniors, starting with your body weight or light weights (2-3lbs) and focusing on good form and technique is best.

Proper stretching and balance exercises can improve flexibility and help prevent falls. Gentle but purposeful movements such as seated leg lifts, hip circles, or single-leg balance can help you maintain good posture and strength.

Aerobic exercises such as dancing, cycling, swimming, or walking can help strengthen the heart, lungs, and circulation. These exercises also provide joint protection and help reduce the risk of obesity and other chronic illnesses.

It's not necessarily about pushing your body to do something that it's not capable of doing. It's more about the concept of *progressive overload*. The more active you are, the better your body will handle specific stresses and routine activities. Over time, as you continuously challenge yourself safely and reasonably, you will improve your capacity to perform various tasks and physical feats.

Step 4: Be More Mindful

Mindfulness is an essential tool for you to use to maintain physical balance as you age. With mindfulness practice, you can better connect with your body, recognize your physical limitations, and manage any age-related pain issues. Mindfulness also provides you with tools to stay mentally and emotionally fit and independent.

One mindfulness technique is body scanning. This technique requires you to pay attention to your entire body, noticing the sensations in each body part. During this practice, you should focus on where your body is touching the ground, the air, and the tension or relaxation experienced in any part of it. This help creates a connection between body and mind that lead to improved physical balance.

Mindful breathing is another valuable technique to connect with your body and improve balance. This practice requires you to focus entirely on your breath, noticing the sensations of inhalation and exhalation. Breathing will assist you in cultivating relaxation and a sense of stillness.

Mindful stretching is also a technique you can practice to stay balanced. It involves focusing on the breath and being aware of any stress or anxiety in the body throughout the movement. Stretching helps to increase flexibility and range of motion while increasing blood flow and reducing tension in the body.

Finally, stress reduction through mindfulness is an essential tool for you to use. Meditation, yoga, and other relaxation techniques are ways to achieve mindfulness. These techniques can help you maintain physical balance and stay healthy. Focusing on the present moment and slowing down the rate of your thoughts can help reduce physical tension in the body. Paying attention to your body and concentrating on relaxation makes you more likely to keep fit, independent, and at peace.

BALANCE EXERCISES

As I've mentioned, our balance can become compromised as we age. Fortunately, a variety of exercises can be used to help improve balance and reduce the risk of falls. This section will discuss some of the most effective activities for improving balance. I will review some exercises focusing on strengthening the core muscles, improving coordination, and increasing flexibility. I will also discuss the importance of proper form and technique when performing these exercises. So let's get started!

Single Leg Balance

Single-leg balance exercises are beneficial as they can help strengthen the lower body muscles, improve balance and coordination, and increase the range of motion in the hip and ankle joints. Additionally, increasing your body's stability can help improve fitness and reduce the risk of falls.

To perform this exercise:

1. Start by standing on two feet, with your arms at your sides and your eyes focused on an immovable point before you.
2. Lift your left foot off the floor and hold it about six inches off the ground for 30 or more seconds and then lower the left foot back to the ground.
3. Balance on your right foot and maintain your posture without moving or bending your knee.

4. Hold the balance for 30 or more seconds and then lower the left foot back to the ground.
5. Repeat the exercise for the opposite leg. You should stand next to a wall if your ability to balance could be stronger.
6. If you can balance for over 40 seconds, increase the time to 60 seconds.
7. When you gain more control, you can exercise longer with your eyes closed.

Tree Pose

The Tree Pose is an excellent exercise because it can help to improve balance and coordination, strengthen the core muscles and lower body, increase flexibility, and reduce stress and anxiety. It can also help improve posture and relieve pain from joint issues such as arthritis and sciatica.

To perform this exercise:

1. Begin by standing comfortably on a flat surface with your feet about hip-width apart.
2. Raise your arms over your head, palms facing down.
3. Begin to bend your right knee and slowly place your right foot up the inside of your left thigh, keeping your toes pointed down.
4. Lift your arms over your head and slowly lower your right elbow onto your right knee.
5. Bring your hands together in front of your chest as if in a prayer position.

6. Focus your gaze on a single point before you when in the pose.
7. Hold the pose for up to a minute before slowly releasing and repeating with the left leg.

Repeat the Tree Pose 2 -3 more times in both directions and make sure to keep your breathing even and focus your gaze on a point in front of you to maintain balance. Again, consistency is key to improving your ability to balance.

Tightrope Walk

No, you will not be walking on an actual tightrope! This walk is great because it improves balance, coordination, and flexibility. This exercise also helps strengthen the core muscle group and can provide a cardio workout if done more vigorously. In addition to the physical benefits, the tightrope walk can help reduce stress and anxiety in seniors.

To perform this exercise:

1. Start by standing with your feet shoulder-width apart, keeping your back straight and your head up.
2. Place your palms flat against your sides and take a slow, controlled step with one foot, keeping your weight balanced over the center of your body.
3. Move slowly, picking up the pace only once you become comfortable with the motion.
4. As you step with one foot, gently move the opposite arm forward, keeping your elbow slightly bent.

5. As you become confident in the motion, you can shift your weight from one side to the other as you move along.
6. Continue walking for about 10-15 steps, then turn around and walk back in the opposite direction.

Repeat this exercise for a few minutes each session. When performing the tightrope walk exercise, it is essential to remember to move slowly and carefully. Stop if you feel any discomfort or pain.

Flamingo Stand

The flamingo stand exercise is an excellent exercise that helps to improve strength and balance in your lower body and core. This exercise engages the core muscles, hips, glutes, legs, and feet to help give the body the stability and support it needs to stay upright. The flamingo stand also helps to improve posture, coordination, and blood flow in the limbs for better overall mobility.

To perform this exercise:

1. Stand near a sturdy wall or chair for support. Place your feet hip-width apart and keep your arms at your sides.
2. Slowly raise one leg off the ground and reach it out in front of you, keeping your hips level and your toes pointed forward.

3. Find your balance and hold the position for 15-30 seconds.
4. Slowly lower your raised leg and switch to the other side.
5. Repeat the exercise 8-10 times on each side.

Lunges

The lunge exercise is one of the best exercises because it can help them improve their balance and core strength while strengthening the major muscles of the legs. It's a low-impact activity that builds up strength and stability simultaneously. The benefits of the lunge exercise include improving coordination, increasing flexibility, promoting better posture and balance, strengthening muscles, and helping prevent falls.

To perform this exercise:

1. Begin by standing with your feet placed hip-width apart and your hands on your hips.
2. Step your right leg forward, keeping your left leg stationary.
3. Bend your right leg and lower your body, ensuring your right knee does not go past your toes.
4. Lower your body until your left knee is just above the floor, keeping your back straight and your head up.
5. Push off with your right foot and step back to your starting position.
6. Repeat with your left leg.
7. Do 10-15 repetitions on each leg.

Make sure to use proper form and body alignment during this exercise. If you need more clarification about your form or if you experience any pain, stop and consult a doctor or physical therapist.

CONCLUSION

In conclusion, maintaining a good balance as we age is important for staying healthy and independent. As you age, your balance system deteriorates, making it even more vital to incorporate balance maintenance into your daily regimens. Regular exercises such as yoga, tai chi, and Pilates improve balance and help you stay fit and active. Furthermore, you should consult a health care professional to ensure that your prior health issues or medications, if any, do not contribute to balance system dysfunction. You can maintain your balance and remain active and independent for life with proper care and nutrition.

3

STRENGTH

S trength is one of the essential elements of overall physical health and wellness—for people of all ages, but particularly for those over fifty-five. Strength training is a form of physical activity that helps you to achieve greater levels of strength, muscle mass, and bone density. It is especially beneficial to those looking to improve their overall health, promote independence and participation in activities, reduce the risk of injury, and manage chronic conditions.

This chapter will explore the concept of strength and why strength training is necessary as we age. I will show you what a sample strength training program looks like and how you can begin to create your own tailored program. This chapter aims to provide you with a foundational knowledge of strength training, allowing you to make informed decisions and pursue activities that better your physical, mental, and emotional well-being. We'll talk about exercises best suited for seniors over 60, the types of equipment and tools available, and the considerations you should consider when setting up your program. We'll also cover safe and proper exercise techniques so that you can make the most out of your strength training sessions.

Strength training requires little or no financial investment to be effective. You can implement it inexpensively and effectively with minimal equipment or funds. There are many ways to work on strength using bodyweight exercises that don't require spending lots of money on equipment. Bodyweight exercises such as push-ups, crunches, and squats can all help build muscle. If weights are necessary, use what is around the house or apartment cans of vegetables, bottled water, etc. Resistance bands are also an excellent and low-cost option to add resistance to bodyweight exercises. Lastly, exercising outdoors using hills, rocks, and uneven surfaces all help improve strength and coordination. With a bit of creative thinking, one can find plenty of ways to work on strength without breaking the bank.

A proper strength training regimen is an excellent way to improve physical health, reduce joint pain, and increase life expectancy. Building muscle can reduce stress on your bones, joints, and connective tissues, leading to improved joint mobility and increased physical activity. Strength training also increases bone density, reducing the risk of osteoporosis and fractures.

Strength training also raises the body's metabolism, improving weight management. This benefits those with arthritis, as excess weight can cause additional stress on the joints and muscles. Joint stability, which reduces the risk of falls and other injuries, is another benefit that strength training can provide.

Finally, strength training helps build physical endurance and stamina, which can improve the overall quality of life. Many engage in strength training and can perform their daily activities with greater ease and longer. This increased activity lifestyle can lead to better health and a longer, healthier life expectancy.

By the end of this chapter, you should have an understanding of strength and why strength training is important. You will have the tools to create and maintain your strength training program that meets your individual needs and goals. Several sample strength training programs will be provided for reference and to get started with. I hope that this chapter encourages and inspires you to pursue strength training and enjoy the many benefits that come with it.

WHAT DO WE MEAN WHEN WE SAY STRENGTH?

Strength is often confused with other forms of fitness, such as power or endurance. Strength training is a great way to increase health, but having a better understanding of what strength actually is and how it differs from other forms of fitness can help you use it more effectively. In this section, I will discuss why it is essential to understand these differences before starting a strength training program, with particular emphasis on those 60 and over. I will share the types of strength, what they each mean, and how strength training can help people of all ages. Finally, explore the benefits of strength training and how it can be used to achieve various fitness goals.

To start, explaining the differences between muscular strength and endurance properly is essential. Muscular strength is the ability of a muscle or muscle group to generate force against resistance. It is the maximum amount of force a muscle or muscle group can generate. Muscular endurance, on the other hand, is the ability of a muscle or muscle group to sustain repeated contractions or continuous force against resistance. It is typically measured by a person's ability to perform a muscular task, such as doing push-ups or squats, for a period of time. In other words, muscular strength is the amount of force a person can exert in one go, while muscular endurance measures the length of time a person can sustain a specific amount of pressure.

Building muscular strength in your body can provide numerous benefits. Regular strength training can help maintain your independence with performing everyday activities. Increasing muscular strength can also improve seniors' overall health and well-being by decreasing their risk of falls, which is a leading cause of injury for individuals over 65. Regular strength training can help you prevent or reduce chronic conditions such as arthritis, osteoporosis, and diabetes since stronger muscles can better withstand damage from disease-causing inflammation. Furthermore, regular strength training can help you maintain your balance, coordination, and coordination of motor skills, which are extremely important for safety and can help reduce the risk of dangerous falls.

Finally, strength training can help you improve your posture, reducing your risk of back pain and providing better support for your body's joints. In addition, older individuals may experience improved moods with regular strength training. Strength training can boost endorphins, which are hormones that are associated with increased energy and lower levels of stress and anxiety. The increased muscular strength achieved through regular strength training can provide numerous benefits, including increased independence, better physical and mental health, enhanced safety, and overall well-being. These are just a sneak peek into the advantages of a consistent strength training program.

Different Tools Used in Strength Training

There are many different kinds of strength training programs and exercises. Anyone can enjoy the benefits of strength training by pursuing an exercise program suitable for them. After all, everyone has a different physiological makeup. Performing particular exercises effectively depends on your experience. That's why a proper strength training program should be tailored for everyone. This section will talk about a few examples of tools used in strength training as you develop your own regimen.

Free weights are weights that move freely, usually manipulated by the user in any way to create resistance and develop strength in the body. A lot of people make use of free weights when doing strength training. The barbell squat is an example of a free-weight exercise in strength training. This exercise involves standing with a barbell loaded with weight on the back of the shoulders, with the feet slightly wider than hip-width apart and the toes pointed slightly outwards. The goal is to squat down, lowering the hips until the thighs parallel the floor, before squeezing the glutes and standing back up to the start position.

Medicine balls and sandbags are training tools used to increase strength, power, and dynamic performance, explicitly targeting the core muscles. Medicine balls typically consist of a weight-filled ball that can be tossed, caught, or lifted during exercises. Sandbags, however, are filled with adjustable straps, handles, or loops, often filled with sand or other matter, depending on their design. Medicine balls and sandbags are excellent tools for performing dynamic exercises that incorporate full-body movements instead of more traditional weight training using dumbbells, barbells, and machines.

An example of a medicine ball or sandbag exercise is the slam. This exercise targets the hips and core. To perform this exercise, stand upright, holding the medicine ball above the head with the feet shoulder-width apart. Slam the medicine ball down onto the ground as hard and pick it up as fast as possible, then return to a standing position with the ball in your hands again, repeating for a fixed period, 30 - 60 seconds, depending on your ability. Don't worry if you do not have a medicine ball. Use a partially deflated ball (basketball, soccer, etc.) For sandbag exercises, an example is the sandbag clean and press. To perform this exercise, start with the sandbag in front of the body, then explosively lift it, bringing it up to shoulder height. Then, press the bag up with the arms until they extend directly overhead. Then, lower the load slowly down to the starting position. This exercise targets the shoulders, upper back, arms, and core. This exercise is similar to the traditional dumbbell clean and press but uses the filled sandbag instead.

Weight machines are an important piece of equipment found in strength training gyms. They provide an isolated exercise for specific muscle groups while using adjustable weight resistance, making them safe and effective for people of all fitness levels. Weight machines target individual muscles through a single compound exercise, which can help improve muscular power, endurance, and flexibility. They use free weights such as dumbbells, barbells and various parts like cables, pulleys, and levers.

An example of a weight machine exercise is a Seated Row. Performed from a seated position, this exercise works the back muscles and helps strengthen the lats, traps, and biceps. The user holds on to two handles connected to the weight machine and pulls them back with an even and controlled motion, keeping their shoulders pulled back and their back straight. The user completes one repetition by returning the handles to their initial position. This exercise can be varied depending on the chosen weight level and the speed of the activity.

Resistance bands are effective tools for strength training, as they provide variable resistance for exercises. The resistance increases with resistance bands as the band is stretched further, giving a more intense workout than free weights. Resistance bands can be used to strengthen almost any major muscle group, and they can also be used to improve balance, range of motion, and coordination in seniors.

To perform the Seated Row exercise using resistance bands, sit on the floor with your feet straight ahead, and hold each end of the resistance band in each hand. Keeping the arms straight, pull your hands towards your chest and hold the position for 3 seconds before returning to the starting position. Depending on your fitness level, 2 - 3 sets of 10-15 repetitions.

Bodyweight exercises are strength training exercises that use only a person's body weight for resistance rather than additional external weight such as dumbbells, kettlebells, weighted bars, or machines. Bodyweight exercises can be great for strengthening the body, as they involve the use of multiple muscle groups at once, such as when doing push-ups, pull-ups, burpees, planks, or squats.

For adults over 60, bodyweight exercises that don't require too much pushing or jumping might include Wall Sits, heel raises, arm circles, and side planks add significant value. Wall Sits involve:

- Standing with your back against a wall.
- Sliding your back down until your thighs are parallel to the ground.
- Holding the position for anywhere from one to two minutes.

Heel raises involve standing with feet hip-width apart and slowly raising your heels as high as possible, holding the position for a few seconds before lowering back down. Arm circles involve standing with your arms outstretched to the sides and rotating them in small circles. Side planks include lying on your side with your feet stacked one on the other, then propping yourself up on your forearm, lifting your hips off the ground, and holding the position. Side planks can be performed against the wall or using a bench.

THE IMPORTANCE OF STRENGTH TRAINING

Discussed already are some different benefits of strength training and why it's important to integrate a fitness routine into any individual's daily life regardless of how old they are. But when it comes to older adults, there's always extra attention on catering to specific needs regarding overall health and wellness. In this section of the book, I will take on a deeper dive into the real benefits of strength training for older adults.

Rebuilding Muscle

Strength training is effective in building and maintaining muscle mass. Resistance training is known to increase both muscle size and strength in seniors. It is especially beneficial for those experiencing sarcopenia; the natural decrease in muscle mass and strength often occurs with aging. Resistance training can increase muscle strength and size, improve mobility, and reduce the risk of falls and fractures. Strength training can also help with balance, coordination, posture, and the ability to perform daily activities.

When strength training, you should begin with lower-intensity exercises such as balance exercises and light resistance training. As your strength and confidence increase, so can the intensity and complexity of the activities. It is important to start slowly and build up power. It is also important to give muscles time to rest between workouts.

Strength training increases muscle size and strength, which can help you remain independent longer. Adding healthier nutrition ensures your body receives the necessary nutrients for muscle growth and repair.

Recharging Metabolism

The vast body of research available in the health and fitness community agrees that strength training is an effective way for seniors to help recharge their metabolism. It is also known as resistance training and can help improve muscular strength, balance, endurance, and metabolism (Buckley, 2020). Metabolism is the process by which the body converts food into energy. As you age, your metabolism begins to slow down, which can lead to weight gain, fatigue, and various health conditions. Strength training can help improve muscle mass and metabolism, leading to better overall health and well-being.

Strength training can help prevent age-related changes in metabolism, such as a slowdown in metabolic rate and a decrease in muscle mass (Vieira, 2019). As a result, it can help prevent a reduction in metabolism, leading to weight gain and fatigue. Strength training can also help increase the body's ability to break down nutrients more efficiently, resulting in improved metabolism and energy (Noakes, 2017).

Strength training can also help reduce the risk of osteoporosis and cardiovascular disease. Research shows that strength training can help increase bone mineral density, reduce inflammation, and improve overall bone health (Villareal et al., 2017). Additionally, strength training can improve cardiovascular health, improving cardiovascular risk factors such as blood pressure, cholesterol, and body fat (Thomas et al., 2018). By helping to recharge your metabolism, strength training can help you enjoy an overall higher quality of life. Live long and strong!

Reducing Fat

Strength training is an effective way to reduce fat and improve overall health for seniors. Studies have shown that strength training is beneficial for reducing body fat in this population. One study found that seniors who engaged in strength training for eight weeks lowered their body fat by 3% (Lage-Oliveira, et al., 2015). It is safe to assume that training for more than eight weeks should yield even better fat-loss results.

A proper strength training program also promotes increased metabolic activity, which requires more energy and aids in burning fat. Research has found that strength training increases the resting metabolic rate, which is the body's energy needed to sustain essential functions (Fano et al., 2014). This means that after completing a strength training session, your body continues to burn more calories than it would have if you did not engage in strength training.

Lastly, strength training can also help to reduce visceral fat, which is located around the internal organs. Visceral fat is associated with many diseases and conditions, including cardiovascular disease and Type II diabetes (Teixeira et al., 2017). By engaging in strength training, you can reduce visceral fat and lower your risk of certain health conditions.

Reducing Resting Blood Pressure

Studies indicate that regular strength training can help seniors improve muscular strength, coordination, and physical conditioning and reduce resting blood pressure. This benefits older adults, who are more likely to suffer from hypertension (high blood pressure).

Research suggests that resistance training can help reduce resting blood pressure by increasing nitric oxide production in the body. Nitric oxide is a gas produced by the endothelium, which plays an important role in controlling blood pressure. By stimulating nitric oxide production, strength training can improve blood vessel flexibility and regulate the dilation and contraction of blood vessels, thus reducing resting blood pressure in seniors (Al-Obaidi et al., 2007).

Strength training can also help lower resting blood pressure by increasing insulin sensitivity, which allows the metabolism to process glucose more effectively. Increased insulin sensitivity reduces resting blood pressure by decreasing the release of hormones (such as aldosterone and angiotensin II) from the adrenal glands and thus decreasing systemic vascular resistance. Furthermore, strength training can help reduce resting blood pressure by promoting weight loss, improving aerobic capacity, and decreasing body fat percentage.

Improving Blood Lipid Profiles

Strength training helps improve blood lipid profiles for older adults by increasing their physical activity and encouraging healthy lifestyle changes. During physical activity, muscles use lipids for energy, increasing fat utilization in the blood. Studies have shown that aerobic and resistance training exercises can reduce total cholesterol, low-density lipoprotein cholesterol (LDL-C), and triglyceride levels while increasing high-density lipoprotein cholesterol (HDL-C) levels. Additionally, strength training increases lipoprotein lipase activity, which helps regulate lipids' metabolism in the blood. Increasing physical activity has also improved insulin sensitivity, decreased triglyceride levels, and enhanced seniors' blood lipid profile (Wilson et al., 2020).

Enhancing Postcoronary Performance

Strength training helps you with postcoronary performance by improving the ability of your heart and circulatory system to transport oxygen, enhancing the efficiency with which the heart and lungs process oxygen, and increasing the body's capacity to use the oxygen that is delivered. These improvements increase energy and strength, endurance, and functional ability.

Consistent strength training can benefit you if you have experienced a cardiac event by improving the circulation and delivery of oxygen to the heart muscle, thus improving the muscle's ability to contract and work effectively. Strength training also increases the heart, lungs, and skeletal muscles' capacity to use this oxygen, thus increasing your overall functional capacity and endurance (Duckworth, 2014). According to Magnani, Laus et al. (2008), conditions that limit the intake and transport of oxygen, such as chronic obstructive pulmonary disease (COPD), can be improved through strength training, while Friedenreich, Thorgeir, et al. (2007) showed that cardiac rehabilitation which includes strength training may reduce the risk of coronary events in coronary artery patients.

Resisting Diabetes

For diabetics or pre-diabetics, having a consistent strength training program has been proven to help resist diabetes by improving their glycemic control, reducing insulin resistance, and improving glucose metabolism (Mustard, Papamichael, & Brawley, 2003). Glycemic control, or maintaining stable and healthy glucose levels, is crucial for reducing the risk of developing diabetes and helping those with diabetes manage their disease. With strength training, glucose metabolism is improved, and insulin resistance is decreased, leading to better glycemic control (Pointon, Talbot, Anderson, & Keogh, 2018).

In addition to improving glycemic control, strength training has been shown to help seniors with diabetes reduce the amount of daily medications required to manage their diabetes

(Xing et al., 2017). A 2019 study found that after only 16 weeks of strength training, seniors with type 2 diabetes experienced a significant decrease in daily medication and improvements in body composition, insulin sensitivity, and physical function (Li, Zhao, Jin, Deng, & Yu, 2019).

Increasing Bone Density

Studies have shown that strength training, when done correctly and with sufficient intensity, can lead to increased bone density in both men and women over 65 (Johannsen et al., 2016). This is critical, as decreased bone density is typical in seniors and can lead to frailty and an increased risk of falls and fractures (Nichols & Sanborn, 2011). Strength training stresses the bone, which causes the bone's cells (osteoblasts and osteoclasts) to break down and rebuild it, thereby leading to increased bone density (Lee & Sivarajan, 2001). Strength training adds value to the prevention of osteoporosis. This is a condition that results in brittle and weak bones.

Decreasing Physical Discomfort

Strength training helps decrease physical discomfort in several ways. Regular strength training helps increase muscle mass and strength for better physical performance, increasing stability and balance (Lauder, 2011). By building strength around joints and supporting structures, older adults can better maintain their occupations and lifestyle activities (Miyajima, Griffiths, & Gaskin, 2011). Additionally, strength training helps reduce the risk of injury by enhancing the body's musculoskeletal system, which decreases joint pain (Yeaw et al., 2020). Regular strength training may also help reduce inflammation in the body, which can further reduce physical discomfort (Truchon, Bélanger, & Llanes, 2015). Finally, strength training helps prevent hormonal changes that occur as part of aging and can cause discomfort (Weatherby & Cox, 2017).

Enhancing Mental Health

Seniors who engage in an active strength training program are likely to benefit from an improved mood and reduced symptoms of stress and depression (Dwivedi et al., 2018). Exercise generally releases endorphins, which are natural hormones responsible for feelings of happiness. Strength training can also help to strengthen the cognitive function and further contribute to improved mental health outcomes. Strength training increases muscle mass, flexibility, and coordination. This allows you to participate in other physical activities more effectively; you feel physically capable and are more likely to participate in activities promoting mental health, such as socialization, creative activities, and volunteerism (Babbie & Mouton, 2020). Overall, strength training is an effective tool to help enhance mental health and well-being.

Reversing Physical Frailty

As they get older, one of the greatest fears of many people is the idea of growing frail and falling. This fear of falling is real. Strength training helps to reverse physical frailty in seniors by increasing muscle mass and strength, improving functional ability, enhancing balance and coordination, improving glycemic control, and decreasing the frailty-related risk of falls.

These exercises strengthen muscle fibers, enabling the muscles to contract more powerfully (McGowan, 2015). This increased power helps with activities of daily living, like walking up steps or reaching up to grab something from a high shelf (McGowan, 2015). Additionally, strength training will help to decrease the risk of osteoporosis, arthritis, diabetes, and cardiovascular disease in older adults (PubMed Health, 2007).

Muscle mass and strength are important aspects of physical frailty as we age. Strength training helps to increase muscle mass and strength, aiding in activities of daily living. Research has found that strength training exercises for seniors, including upper and lower body movements, multiple planes of motion, and short rest intervals, increase muscle strength and aid in reversing physical frailty (Hagerman, et al., 2018). Regular strength training also helps to improve functional ability in seniors with physical weakness, helping them become more independent with activities of daily living. Research has found that strength training improves physical function, with improvements in both upper and lower body muscle strength (Rantanen, et al., 1998).

HOW STRENGTH TRAINING HELPS TREAT CHRONIC DISEASES

Strength training is a critical aspect of any health and wellness plan. As you age, your muscles do not regenerate strength and stamina as quickly as they used to—making strength training a key part of any health regime. But did you know that strength training has also been shown to provide health benefits beyond simple tools for physical fitness? Researchers have discovered that strength training can help address certain chronic diseases, especially in seniors.

Cancer

Cancer is a severe chronic disease that poses a significant health risk to older populations. According to the World Health Organization, cancer is the second most common cause of death among adults aged 65 and over, accounting for over 11 million deaths worldwide in 2020 (World Health Organization, 2021).

This increased prevalence in older adults is due to the normal aging process, which causes damage to the body's cells. It increases the chances of developing genetic mutations linked to cancer and other risk factors, including a sedentary lifestyle and other potential environmental or lifestyle-related causes (Cancer.net, 2020).

Strength training, which uses resistance to increase muscle strength, has been suggested to be potentially beneficial for elderly individuals to reduce their risk of developing cancer. It helps keep your body strong, which in turn helps your body's immune system fight off cancer cells. Strength training has also been proven to help reduce the risks of developing other chronic diseases that are more common among the elderly, such as heart disease and diabetes (Miller et al., 2017). Furthermore, studies have found that strength training can reduce the risk of all-cause mortality among older adults and improve the overall quality of life (Konzelmann et al., 2020).

Cardiovascular Disease

Cardiovascular disease (CVD), particularly prevalent in older adults, is considered the largest single cause of death world-wide, accounting for over a third of all deaths in adults over 65 (Kasza et al., 2007). There is a range of diseases that affect the heart, including coronary heart disease, stroke, congestive heart failure, and peripheral arterial disease (Yeh & Haskell, 2008). These diseases detrimentally affect survival, quality of life, physical functioning, and mental health (Kasza et al., 2007).

Strength training has been proposed as an effective exercise to combat CVD in elderly populations. It has been demonstrated to reduce resting heart rate and blood pressure, promote weight loss and healthy blood cholesterol levels, and improve overall muscular strength and endurance (Yeh & Haskell, 2008).

Strength training has emerged as an effective form of exercise to reduce the risk of CVD in elderly populations, potentially improving seniors' health and quality of life.

Obesity

Older adults are particularly vulnerable to the adverse health effects of severe obesity, which can lead to numerous chronic illnesses such as type 2 diabetes, cardiovascular disease, stroke, hypertension, and certain types of cancer. This health condition often results from a lack of physical activity, poor lifestyle choices, or aging changes in metabolism.

Strength training is an efficient and effective tool to combat severe obesity among older adults. Through strength training, older individuals can increase their level of physical activity, helping to build muscle which in turn helps to reduce fat mass. This helps to lower blood pressure and improve blood sugar levels. Furthermore, engaging in strength training can help to improve joint and bone strength, reduce the risk of falls, and improve overall balance and coordination. Paired with good nutrition, an aging individual can improve their chances of living a long and healthy life without illness complications.

To experience maximum benefits from strength training, focus on techniques involving large and small muscle groups and use free weights, resistance bands, bodyweight exercises, and machines. Additionally, interval training and circuit training techniques provide a potentially more significant challenge that can further improve metabolic rates.

Regular physical activity—including strength training—is an important component of any lifestyle for promoting better overall health and combating severe obesity. However, it is important to remember that safe and effective strength training programs should always be tailored to your skill level and physical condition.

Type 2 Diabetes

Type 2 diabetes is a serious and chronic condition, especially among seniors. As of 2021, over 35 million people aged 65 years and older in the US are living with this metabolic disorder (American Psychology Association, 2021). This type of diabetes is caused by a combination of hundreds of genes and lifestyle factors, such as physical inactivity, poor diet, and excess weight, which are more common as individuals age.

Those with type 2 diabetes are at increased risk of developing a wide array of health problems, such as heart disease, stroke, vision loss, foot problems, nerve damage, and kidney damage (American Diabetes Association, 2021). Therefore, this disorder significantly lowers the quality of life and increases the risk of death in seniors (American Psychology Association, 2021).

Strength training is a powerful tool to help those with type 2 diabetes to improve their metabolic health, body composition, and overall physical health. Studies have shown that strength training can reduce insulin resistance and lower fasting glucose levels. This is partly because resistance training helps increase skeletal muscle mass and the muscles' capacity to metabolize glucose (American Psychology Association, 2021). Additionally, strength training can increase metabolic rate and reduce body fat, limiting the burden of type 2 diabetes on the body (American Psychology Association, 2021).

For the most part, engaging in strength training is a reliable way to help those with type 2 diabetes lower their risk and manage their symptoms. It is important to talk to the doctor and follow a tailored program based on your individual health, needs, and goals.

STRENGTH TRAINING EXERCISES

Earlier, I mentioned that a lack of financial resources shouldn't have to be a roadblock to staying fit even as you age. If you have the resources to buy fancy gym equipment or pay for a basic gym membership, that's good. If you already have access to a private coach or a training facility that will allow you to stay in shape, then you should definitely make the most out of these resources. But just because you don't have a nice fancy weight machine or a set of dumbbells doesn't mean you can't get fit. In this section of the chapter, I will share with you some simple exercises you can do without using expensive gym equipment, the benefits of each exercise, and how you can execute them safely. Please consult your physician before you begin. Finally, listen to your body and move only as far as is comfortable and with no pain. Dominate your health!

Lying Hip Bridges

Overall we spend a significant amount of time sitting. The lying hip bridge exercise is a great exercise for seniors as it is low impact and can help to improve glute strength, mobility, and balance. The exercise helps improve strength and stability in the front and back of the lower body, reducing the risk of falls and other injuries. It also helps to improve posture and promote proper body alignment.

To perform this exercise:

1. Begin by lying on your back with your knees bent and your feet flat on the ground. Your arms should be by your sides.
2. Engaging your core, press your feet into the ground and lift your hips off the ground. Try to align your feet, knees, and hips so that your body creates a straight line from the shoulders to the knees.
3. Hold the bridge position for five to ten seconds, then lower your hips back to the ground.
4. Repeat for a total of 10 repetitions.

Once you have become comfortable with this exercise, you can progress to performing the bridge with one leg at a time. Balance can be further challenged by performing the bridges on an uneven or unstable surface.

Squats to Chair

As the years go by, fully functioning legs become a must-have. You will need to get up and sit down, walk up and down stairs, and bend down to pick things up. The Squats to Chair exercise is a great, low-impact exercise that can help strengthen the lower body and improve balance and coordination. It's an excellent choice for seniors who want to stay active and independent, especially in the bathroom. One exercise can make a difference. Squats are that exercise.

To perform this exercise:

1. Stand with your back against a wall or chair for support. Keep your feet shoulder-width apart, toes pointing slightly outward.
2. Slowly bend your knees until your thighs parallel the floor.
3. Hold that posture for a few seconds, then slowly rise.
4. Repeat this 10-15 times.

Although this is a simple exercise, keeping your posture and moving slowly and steadily is essential. If you feel too much strain, stop and rest. Gradually increase the number of repetitions as your strength and stamina increase.

Wall Push-Ups

Wall push-ups are excellent exercises for you to improve strength and stability. Wall push-ups are similar to regular push-ups. However, they can be performed directly against a wall eliminating the floor. This makes the exercise ideal for those 60 and over, as it is less taxing than traditional push-ups.

Benefits include improved strength and stability and increased range of motion due to the static position. Improved balance and posture can also be achieved as the wall provides stability and support.

To perform this exercise:

1. Stand facing a wall, with your feet slightly wider than shoulder-width apart.
2. Lean into the wall and place your hands on the wall at the same height as your shoulders. The elbows should be slightly bent.
3. Push away from the wall, keeping your back and body straight.
4. Lower the chest towards the wall and press back up, keeping proper form. Keep the elbows close to the body while pushing away from the wall.

Performing three sets of 8-12 push-ups are recommended. The exercise should be done at a pace that is comfortable and manageable. To maximize the benefits, you should be mindful of your form and technique.

Side Lying Circles

The Side Lying Circles exercise is an excellent way to improve balance and posture in seniors. Additionally, it helps to strengthen the core muscles and maintain flexibility. Furthermore, this exercise can be done in the comfort and privacy of the home, making it an accessible and enjoyable form of exercise. It can be done while lying on a soft surface such as a mat or carpet, and it helps to strengthen the core and low back muscles while promoting flexibility and mobility.

To perform this exercise:

1. Begin by lying on your side, with your knees bent slightly and your hips stacked.
2. Then lift your top leg up and gently move it in a circular motion across your body. Keep your leg close to the body and move forward and backward in a small range of motion.
3. You should move your leg in a clockwise direction for 10-15 repetitions before switching to a counterclockwise rotation for 10-15 repetitions.

Quadruped Opposite Arm and Leg Balance

The quadruped opposite arm and leg balance exercise is an effective way to promote core strength and mobility. The exercise requires you to maintain a stable position while balancing on your hands and knees. This activity helps strengthen and stabilize the abdominals and the back and legs.

To perform this exercise:

1. Begin on your hands and knees with the spine in a neutral position.
2. Keep your head in line with your spine. Do not let it tilt forward.
3. Slowly lift the left hand and right foot off the ground and hold in a straight line.
4. Return to the start position, and repeat the movement with the right hand and left foot.

5. Complete 10 to 12 repetitions, then switch sides and repeat.
6. Keep your abdominals engaged and your back and legs stable as you perform the exercise.
7. Take slow, controlled movements and avoid any jerky movements.
8. After the exercise, take a few seconds to relax and breathe before performing another set.

Deadbugs

Deadbugs offer a lower risk of injury. It is an easy-to-do, practical, and functional exercise designed to strengthen the core. Deadbugs can also help improve breathing by strengthening the respiratory muscles, allowing one to stay active longer.

To perform this exercise:

1. Start by lying on the floor or the exercise mat. Place your arms in the air, bend your knees, and elevate your feet off the ground.
2. Keeping your lower back on the floor, extend one leg straight, keeping your back stable. Make sure that you keep your abdominal muscles contracted throughout the exercise. Do not arch your back as you extend your leg.
3. Return your leg to the starting position and repeat the movement with the other leg.

4. Once comfortable with both movements, you can increase the difficulty by extending alternating arms and legs simultaneously.
5. Repeat this movement for 8 - 10 repetitions for 2-3 sets.

Keep your back in contact with the floor at all times to ensure you don't put too much strain on your lower back. Do not arch your back as you extend your leg. It is also important to not overextend your legs and that your abdominal muscles remain contracted throughout the exercise.

Side Planks

The side plank is an excellent exercise because it helps maintain core strength, balance, and stability. It works out the muscles of your trunk, hips, legs, arms, shoulders, and neck. It is very challenging with great benefits. If you are a beginner, try the modified version first when you have masters that proceed to the traditional side plank if possible. It's important to note that you should not hold your breath while doing the side plank. Maintain good form to avoid injury. If the exercise causes pain or discomfort, you should stop and consult with your doctor before continuing.

To perform this exercise:

1. Begin by lying on your left side with your elbow bent and directly beneath your shoulder, your legs straight and stacked on each other.
2. Raise your torso and legs off the ground, ensuring your torso is straight and in line with your hips. If your balance is an issue, modify this exercise by placing the top leg bent in front of you. The side closest to the ground will remain straight.
3. Keep your abdominals tight, squeeze your belly button towards your spine, and breathe.
4. Hold the position for 20 - 30 seconds, or as long as you can, then slowly relax as you lower your body back to the ground/floor.
5. Repeat on the other side. Repeat 1 - 2 times, alternating sides.

Wall / Floor Angles

Wall / Floor Angles are a simple, safe, therapeutic exercise that can help you improve your physical posture and mental functioning. This exercise combines traditional resistance strength and endurance benefits with mental stimulation and coordination. Wall/Floor Angles are an easy and effective way for older adults to strengthen their upper bodies. This exercise is beneficial because it helps develop muscular strength, but it also helps improve posture, joint stability, and range of motion. This exercise consists of performing a wall press with your entire back and arms while slowly and methodically gliding along the wall with your arms.

To perform this exercise:

1. Begin by standing with your back and shoulders flat against the wall. Keep your feet shoulder-width apart, and
2. Extend your arms straight above your head, flat against a wall. Palms face out.
3. Holding your back against the wall, slowly glide your arms down the wall just below the shoulders (45-degree angle) perpendicular to the ground
4. Hold for 1 -3 seconds and slowly glide your arms straight back up.
5. Repeat the exercise 8-10 times the routine three times per week. Be sure to breathe deeply throughout the movement.

Floor Angles, the same exercise, is done on the floor. Move your arm as if they were against the wall. Now, move your arms just like on the wall:

1. Lay with your back and back of your hands against the floor and knees bent. Your spine should be as straight as possible.
2. Extend your arms straight above your head, resting on the floor.

3. Squeeze your upper back muscles, slowly gliding your arms below your shoulders to form 45-degree angles perpendicular to the ground.
4. Hold for 1 - 3 seconds.
5. Glide your arms slowly back up straight above your head and repeat 8-10 times the routine three times per week. Be sure to breathe deeply throughout the movement.

Moving slowly and avoiding jerky or sudden movements is an additional safety tip. Also, keep your back and head flat against the wall or floor throughout the exercise. Finally, listen to your body and move only as far as is comfortable and with minimal discomfort.

Pec Stretches

The Pec Stretch is an effective stretching exercise to improve posture, decrease chest muscle tension, and increase chest and shoulder flexibility. This exercise is particularly beneficial for older adults, as it can help to decrease age-related posture deterioration, reduce shoulder and chest pain, and improve mobility.

To perform this exercise:

1. Stand straight with your feet shoulder-width apart and your arms at your sides.
2. Take a deep breath and, while exhaling, reach both arms out in front of you at shoulder height with your palms facing down.
3. Slowly lean forward and exhale, feeling the stretch in your chest muscles as you reach outward.
4. Take 3-5 deep breaths and focus on keeping your chest open to ensure that you are stretching correctly.
5. Slowly return to the starting position and repeat the stretch two or three more times.

Standing Balance

The Standing Balance exercise is an excellent way for seniors to improve their balance and coordination. Additionally, the movement maintains muscle tone and can benefit those suffering from muscular pain or stiffness. The exercise requires one to stand with feet together and arms outstretched. It can be performed with or without the assistance of a wall or chair to help maintain balance.

To perform this exercise:

1. Find a sturdy chair or surface that provides a secure base for the exercise.
2. Stand with your feet about hip-width apart in a comfortable stance. Ensure you have a good posture with your chest and shoulders aligned with your hips.
3. With your arms relaxed at your sides, slowly lift one foot off the ground and hold it for 10-30 seconds. If you can, keep your foot straight or flex it slightly, keeping your toes pointed forward.
4. Return your foot to the floor and change sides, repeating the exercise.
5. As you become more proficient with the exercise, you can increase the time and repetitions to challenge your balance.

Chin Up (At All Times!)

Maintaining good posture is essential for physical and mental well-being, especially for seniors. Keeping one's chin up is vital in keeping the body in alignment, as the alignment of the head, torso, and limbs are connected and contribute to their overall posture. When the chin is kept up, the spine is better aligned, promoting better support of the body, better balance, and improved mobility.

When our posture is not good, the body is out of balance, leading to pain and discomfort. Additionally, slouching can lead to poor circulation, which reduces oxygen flow to the body's muscles, potentially resulting in loss of range of motion and joint pain. Therefore, keeping the chin up is essential for helping to maintain a healthy posture and help avoid these types of issues.

Keeping the chin up also helps to maintain proper breathing and aids in digestion. When the chin is kept up, the chest opens up, allowing for more efficient breathing, which can help contribute to better overall health. Additionally, when the chin is kept up, the stomach is lifted, increasing the effectiveness of digestion and reducing stress on the digestive system.

Finally, good posture can also promote better mental wellness. When the chin is kept up, the body looks taller and straighter, which can impact self-confidence and self-esteem. Good posture can also aid in improving overall mood, as this could potentially reduce feelings of anxiety and depression.

CONCLUSION

In conclusion, strength is crucial to maintaining good health and an active lifestyle. Strength training is essential to maintain strength and muscle mass, reduce the risk of injury and chronic health conditions, and improve overall well-being. With the wide variety of strength exercises and training programs available, you can create a safe and effective routine to meet your individual needs. With commitment, consistency, and patience, you can improve your overall strength and reap the rewards of living a healthy, active, and independent lifestyle.

4

FEARS AND FRUSTRATIONS

I t is okay if you are not okay with aging. Fears and frustrations are a part of life. What are you going to do about it? We all have specific fears and insecurities that make us afraid, especially at 60+. I know you haven't come this far in life without overcoming a lot. You are already strong enough to proceed. You cannot change the past. Your future is an ocean filled with possibilities. Decide and commit to a healthier lifestyle. I am encouraging you to step out of FEAR and into FREEDOM. You can still be healthy and active in the years ahead. The person you will be 3-6 months from now will be celebrating the present you for having the courage to start this journey. Over time, with resilience and consistency, you will find yourself reaching new milestones. Better health and well-being are waiting for you.

Exercising and working out at an older age can seem daunting, but it can also be gratifying. Our bodies start to change as we age, but we can still stay physically active and healthy. Exercise helps promote better physical and mental health, even at age 60 or more.

It can be hard to take the first step, especially when we aren't used to exercising or haven't been active. That's why it's important to take things slowly and gradually. A Peruvian proverb says, "Little by Little, one travels far." Start by doing simple activities like walking inside or outside as much as possible, stretching, and light resistance exercises; if you can, try to find a friend or family member to join the exercise routine. That way, you can motivate each other.

Even the most minor changes can make a significant impact over time. For example, instead of using the elevator, try using the stairs a few times, or add a few minutes of walking or a few extra repetitions to your workout routine. Park farther away in the parking lot. Take a few laps around your home. It's all about taking small, manageable steps each day and building from there.

Find an activity that you enjoy that can help make exercising more fun. These can include dancing, biking, swimming, or gardening. Every action counts, no matter how small.

Focusing on the positive changes that exercise can bring to your life can be a great source of motivation. Exercise has been proven to help boost energy levels, reduce depression, reduce stress, and improve sleep quality. It's never too late to get moving.

Regular exercise is a crucial component of maintaining a healthier lifestyle. Taking the time to work out consistently will strengthen your mind, body, and spirit. Adding a little dedication and effort, you can achieve emotional, physical, and mental accomplishments at any age. Be proud of yourself, and stay active.

AGING - WHAT YOU ARE UP AGAINST

As people age, holding onto physical activity and maintaining an overall fit body can be increasingly challenging. Besides having more physical limitations that may inhibit regular motion, they can encounter other fears and challenges that influence the decision to remain active. In this section, I will explore the various concerns and barriers that many adults 60 and over can face when it comes to physical activity and how they can protect themselves to become more active despite these fears.

Self-Efficacy

Self-efficacy is an individual's belief in their abilities to complete a task or reach a goal. For older adults, self-efficacy may be a barrier to exercise and working out due to the fear of failing or being unable to perform specific activities successfully. This fear may be due to physical limitations associated with aging or concerns about health. They may also feel intimidated by images of young, fit people in fitness magazines or exercising in the gym. This can lead to feelings of low self-esteem and an inability to pursue an exercise program.

Additionally, physical inactivity can lead to various health issues, further decreasing self-efficacy and increasing fear of exercising. It can also make someone more prone to depression, anxiety, and other negative emotions. Therefore, you must encourage yourself by seeking and using available resources and support to help you reach your fitness goals. That is why I wrote this book.

Fear of Injury

Injury is a significant concern for adults at any age regarding exercise and working out. Many seniors aged 65 and over experience an increased risk of injury due to a decline in strength, balance, and coordination as they age. These factors and age-related health problems can make performing specific exercises safely and correctly tricky. However, remember that exercising and keeping active are integral to healthy aging and should not be feared. The key to working out and exercising safely is to start slowly and progress gradually.

Inertia

Inertia can be a severe obstacle to older adults looking to begin a fitness journey due to their fear of the unknown. By the time most people reach their senior years, they've typically become accustomed to the same routines and habits. However, making a change and starting a new exercise regimen can be challenging without any recent experience. The body's resistance to any rapid change due to an inactive lifestyle may cause you to hesitate out of fear that you cannot keep up and will cause injury or harm. Again, the key to achieving your health and wellness goal is to start slow and be consistent.

Depression and Anxiety

Depression and anxiety can be challenging for adults over 60 when starting and maintaining a fitness routine. Many older adults who suffer from depression or anxiety may struggle to find the motivation to engage in physical activities. The most straightforward exercise can appear daunting and overwhelming, especially if they already feel overwhelmed by their mental health symptoms. Others may worry about their physical limitations or the risk of injury, making them hesitant to exercise. In addition, a lack of social support and understanding can make it even more difficult. Despite these difficulties, you must prioritize getting healthier with good nutrition and consistent exercise. This can improve both mental and physical health over time. Be sure to consult your physician. If you are computer savvy, many free resources on YouTube or Facebook can and will add value to your process. Check it out. Join an exercise for the senior group. In this technological age, seeking professional help and advice to help you work out safely and comfortably is not difficult. You have to take that first step.

Self-Conscious

Self-consciousness can be a major challenge for anyone, especially older adults, to exercise. When someone is self-conscious about their physical abilities or appearance, they may feel too embarrassed or scared to go to a gym. Additionally, the fear of making a mistake or being judged by others may discourage them from attempting activities they are not comfortable with. This can lead to avoidance of exercise altogether, which can be detrimental to a person's overall health. You can work out at home or join a group online to combat this barrier. Gather the support and encouragement of family and or friends. Seek more inviting exercise environments and activities designed specifically for people your age.

Health Problems

Health problems can be a significant barrier for older adults regarding exercise. Some health problems that can directly hinder physical activity include chronic conditions such as heart disease, joint pain, and stroke. These conditions can cause pain and difficulty performing physical activity, making it difficult to stay active. Other physical issues, such as poor balance and decreased flexibility, can make it difficult to participate in activities. Mental health can also play a role, as some older people may suffer from depression, which can sap their energy and make it difficult to find the motivation to exercise.

Medications can also be a barrier; some can cause adverse side effects such as increased fatigue or dizziness. Health issues can present formidable obstacles to the elderly regarding participating in and maintaining regular physical activity. You can use exercise modifications or alternatives to help overcome those issues. Try incorporating natural foods, juices, fruits, and spices. This may assist you in lessening or eliminating your dependency on certain prescription medications over time.

Your current health condition will improve with a healthier nutrition and exercise lifestyle. I share more about the benefits of including spices in your diet in my book "Life! Spice It Up!: How To Heal And Transform With 5 Everyday Spices."

Lack of Time

A lack of time can be a substantial hurdle for anyone to exercise and work out. Hopefully, by age 60, you will be retired or nearing retirement and have a more flexible schedule. People who identify as seniors often have other obligations, such as healthcare appointments or caring for family members, that can take up a lot of their time. Additionally, those who struggle with mobility may find they cannot get to and from a gym or fitness class. Here is where establishing and maintaining a home base exercise routine will add tremendous value.

Furthermore, older individuals might need help with energy levels that can prevent them from motivating themselves to work out regularly. There are ways around every barrier. If you genuinely want to live a longer, more robust life.

Lack of Knowledge

Knowledge about exercise or the correct exercise method may be a real challenge. Too much activity can harm specific individuals, and having enough information about how hard to push oneself or which exercises are best can be difficult. You may also have physical limitations and need help understanding how to modify exercises to make them safer. They may be at risk of injury or overexertion without the correct information. Additionally, you may need access to appropriate exercise equipment and facilities, making finding the right resources to work out challenging. There are excellent tutorials online. Instagram, Facebook, and YouTube will be of assistance to you.

Lack of Support

Getting enough support can be a significant discouragement when exercising and working out. Friends, family, and medical professionals can play important roles in encouraging a healthier lifestyle. Without a supportive environment, you may not be motivated to exercise, have difficulty trying new activities, and lose interest in maintaining physical activity without the backing of your community and the ability to access resources. Those above 60 could be more prone to inactivity and associated health problems. There is a time when you will have to encourage yourself! Set a personal goal and achieve it.

Expenses

Seniors may be afraid to start working out because of its high costs. Fitness classes, gym memberships, equipment and supplies, and clothing can all add up quickly for those on a fixed budget. Additionally, older adults may worry about the physical risks of exercise if their bodies aren't used to it and the potential for injury if they haven't been exercising regularly. This thinking is understandable. Therefore, working out from home, online, or in a community center offering free classes is the best option. There are full workout videos for everything at no charge on the internet. YouTube, for example, is a valuable and FREE resource.

COMMON HEALTH CONDITIONS

Exercise plays a vital role in keeping us healthy and fit as we age, but for some seniors, physical limitations or health conditions can hinder staying active. In this section, I'll explore these potential health concerns and, later on, discuss ways to make exercise safer for you. It is strongly suggested that you consult your physician before you begin exercising.

Arthritis

Arthritis can make older people afraid of exercising due to the increased pain and discomfort it may cause. Because the body is not used to the strain exercise places on the joints, the pain could worsen, and the senior may be afraid of this. People with arthritis often experience joint pain and stiffness, making it difficult and uncomfortable to move around. Additionally, the fear of worsening their arthritis can also deter exercise. Start slow and purposeful with your movements. You may choose not to use weights. That is fine. Body-weighted activities shared in Chapter 1 will help you.

Heart Disease

Heart disease can make older adults apprehensive about exercising because of the risk of worsening symptoms or a potential heart attack. Even if the symptoms are mild, exercising could increase heart rate, difficulty breathing, and other symptoms. This fear of exercising can lead to feelings of isolation and depression. However, reduced physical activity can exacerbate heart disease by lowering cardiovascular fitness. Therefore, anyone with heart disease must speak with a doctor before starting any low-impact or high-intensity exercise program. Cycling, aerobics, walking, swimming, and yoga, are just a few of the exercises that can promote heart health by helping to lower blood pressure, reduce inflammation, slow or stop diabetes, and increase muscle strength.

Cancer

Cancer can present a severe challenge for people 60 and over looking to begin an exercise program. Treatment and recovery from cancer can leave one weak and exhausted, and surgeries and chemotherapy can often cause side effects that limit mobility. Additionally, recovering from cancer can be a long process, and intense exercise can negatively affect recovery without proper guidance and care. It is essential for those dealing with cancer to start with low-intensity exercises under medical supervision to ensure they are not putting their body or recovery at risk. Organic foods, herbs, and spices also provide key nutritional benefits that will assist in healing and improved recovery.

Respiratory Disease

Respiratory diseases such as asthma and chronic obstructive pulmonary disease (COPD) can often challenge many over age

60 who want to start exercising. These respiratory diseases can cause breathing difficulties and increased mucus production, ultimately reducing lung function capacity and exercise tolerance. A proper plan should include appropriate breathing exercises and adequate breaks not to overstress the breathing muscles. Additionally, doctors may advise patients to use an inhaler or medication before, during, or after the exercise.

Alzheimer's Disease

Alzheimer's disease (AD) is a progressive, degenerative neurological disorder that can significantly impair an individual's cognitive abilities and disrupt their daily functioning, making it difficult to engage in physical activity. This can be especially true in individuals who may have once been physically active before their diagnosis. As the disease progresses, short-term memory can be significantly affected, making it difficult for those with Alzheimer's disease to remember instructions and be able to engage in physical activities safely.

Additionally, those with this disease may struggle to concentrate for long periods, making sustaining their attention during physical activity strenuous. Alzheimer's disease can also cause changes in mood, behavior, and energy level, making it difficult for elderly individuals with the disorder to find the motivation to engage in physical activity.

Osteoporosis

Osteoporosis can be a major impediment to some people 60 and over who want to start working out, as it can make certain activities, such as weight-bearing exercises, too risky due to a greater chance of fracture. Any weight-bearing activities should be modified to consider existing bone density levels and provide extra support to protect bones from fracture. Chair and other low-impact exercises such as swimming, water aerobics, and biking can provide some of the same health benefits with reduced fracture risk.

Diabetes

For older adults with diabetes, exercise can be a challenge but can offer significant benefits. It can be difficult for them to balance adequate exercise and not overdo it. High-intensity activities may also be strenuous, as older adults with diabetes may not be able to handle the strain, and their blood sugar levels may rise too high. Additionally, they may experience low blood sugar during exercise and need to be able to regularly check and monitor their glucose levels to ensure they don't end up in a dangerous situation. All these considerations can make exercise inconvenient and difficult for seniors with diabetes. If you have diabetes, you must thoroughly warm up and cool down after activity to help prevent strain on your muscles and joints. Regular exercise can cause your body to respond better to insulin, help control your blood sugar levels and reduce risks of heart disease.

Falls

Falls can significantly impact older people's ability to exercise and stay active. As people age, the risk for falls increases, which can be exacerbated by poor vision, impaired balance and coordination, and weakened strength. Falls can cause severe injury and majorly deter those wanting to stay active. Medications designed to increase balance and coordination in older adults can cause dizziness and increase their risk of falls and other side effects.

Some seniors are scared of falling while exercising, which can prevent them from staying active. Therefore, fall prevention measures are essential for any older person who wishes to participate in exercise or other physical activity. Some exercises can be completed effectively from a seated or lying position. These can help strengthen your core and legs until your balance is restored.

Obesity

Obesity can be a considerable obstacle for older adults when engaging in regular physical activity. Obesity increases the risk of many health conditions, making staying active more difficult. As the body ages, joints and muscles become stiffer, and the ability to move around can be diminished. When the body has to carry around extra weight from obesity, it can mean more strain and pain on these joints, resulting in discomfort and an overall decrease in mobility. This can make engaging in activities such as running or even walking difficult, which would be essential parts of a physical activity plan. Additionally, the risk of falls increases with increased body weight, leading to further mobility issues and even physical injuries. In extreme cases, obesity could even lead to the need for full or partial joint replacements, which may make it difficult or even impossible to stay active.

It would be best to consistently incorporate a healthier, more nutritional diet to lose weight. Eighty percent of your weight loss will directly result from the amount of calories you consume. To lose weight, you must establish and maintain a low-calorie diet. This does not mean starving yourself. Many foods you can eat will help you lose weight and not go hungry.

Food Insecurity

Your economic limitations can drastically limit access to healthier foods and available exercise opportunities. This can be due to factors such as limited food options in the area in which you live, lack of access to physical activity recreation or fitness centers, as well as a lack of financial resources to buy equipment or join fitness clubs/programs. This should be easy, as discussed in earlier chapters. Additionally, impoverished seniors may need help to afford healthier and nutrient-dense diets, so their physical activity capabilities are further hindered. This can prevent seniors from getting exercise regularly, leading to health complications. Having limited accessibility and affordability of good nutrition, physical activity, and exercise can seriously impede the overall health and well-being of older individuals living in poverty. Fortunately, it's still possible to maintain a fit and healthy lifestyle without having to spend too much money on gym equipment or memberships. This book is well-equipped to help you find a training program that you can stick to without having to pay anything.

HERE IS WHAT YOU'RE MISSING

As we age, physical activity becomes increasingly important to our overall health and well-being. Not only can regular exercise prevent conditions such as heart disease and osteoporosis, but it can also help improve physical strength, flexibility, and balance. Unfortunately, many older people choose not to exercise and consequently miss out on the numerous benefits that come with a regular exercise regimen. Exercise is therapeutic on many levels.

Improved Mental Health

Exercising and working out can be incredibly beneficial for seniors seeking improved mental health. Staying physically active through regular exercise helps to reduce the level of cortisol (a powerful stress hormone) in the body. This can help seniors to manage daily stressors better, relieve tension and improve overall mental well-being.

Decreased Risk of Falls

Exercise and physical activity are essential elements of an overall strategy to help seniors reduce the risk of falling. Regular physical activity such as walking or muscle-strengthening activities can help improve balance, coordination, muscle strength, and flexibility. Exercise can also help seniors maintain a healthy weight, which can reduce the likelihood of falls and injury. Balance-focused activities such as tai chi, yoga, or other exercise classes can help seniors improve their balance and coordination while also increasing movement and muscle strength, and flexibility. Additionally, strength training helps strengthen the muscles, especially in the legs and abdomen, which can help with balance and the ability to stay active.

Social Engagement

Exercising is vital for seniors to stay active and healthy, but it can also be beneficial for having more social engagement. Regular physical activity helps maintain strength, flexibility, balance, and overall health. However, it can also help boost confidence and provide a sense of community. Exercise can help seniors feel more connected to others, including their peers, as they age. It can empower you to be more courageous and participate in more experiences outside the home.

Improved Brain Function

Studies have shown that aerobic exercises, such as walking or swimming, can increase hippocampal volume, a core area in the brain responsible for new memories, learning, and emotions. The hippocampus also experiences a natural age-related decline, so exercising can help to slow or prevent this decline. Exercising has also been shown to help with the formation of new memories, learning, and also the reversing of cognitive decline. In addition to this, increasing blood and oxygen flow to the brain can help reduce inflammation, and aid in the release of important neurotransmitters like dopamine, helping improve mood and focus.

HOW TO OVERCOME FEARS AND FRUSTRATIONS

As you move forward along your life's journey, you may find yourself feeling tired or out of shape, wishing that you could get stronger, look better, and enjoy yourself and your family more. This book section is here to help you do just that: it will provide you with valuable information and support to help you safely overcome the fears and frustrations of starting an exercise routine. It's time to take charge of your health and feel better—mentally, physically, and emotionally. You will also find motivation and encouragement in my book *Down 100 Pounds: How I Used Positive Affirmations To Transform My Mind & Help Maximize My Weight Loss*. Let's get active, have fun, and build a stronger, healthier you.

Consult Your Physician

It is always wise to consult their physician or healthcare provider before beginning any new type of exercise routine. Because as we age, it is common for our bodies to undergo changes that can make certain kinds of exercise unsafe or less effective. For instance, changes in balance, flexibility, strength, heart rate, and other factors can all indicate a need for modifications in an exercise routine. When starting an exercise program, physicians can evaluate if there are any health problems that would require additional caution and provide advice on how to approach exercise safely and effectively. Additionally, physicians can review medications and other health conditions, such as a history of stroke, heart movements, or osteoporosis, that could increase the risk of exercise. In time, the positive results from your nutrition and fitness transformation may cause the elimination or reduction of some medications. Therefore, consulting a doctor or physician throughout your journey is essential to ensure safety and health benefits when beginning an exercise routine.

Schedule Your Workouts

Older adults should schedule their workouts in order to stay consistent because it provides them with a certain level of accountability. When an appointment for training is carved into your schedule, you're more likely to stick to it than when you're just relying on yourself to remember to work out. Split scheduling also allows you to break your workouts down into manageable chunks. You could break up your exercise into brief but consistent mini-sessions if you have limited time, energy, or mobility. Working out at a regular time each day gives your body a chance to rest and recover in between. It also encourages people to exercise more frequently, which can help prevent age-related diseases, such as arthritis, and make overall life more enjoyable. Scheduling your workouts will also help ensure that you're doing your best to make progress. It's easy to get distracted by day-to-day tasks, but when you have a plan and a schedule, you're more likely to stay on track and see actual progress.

Perform Mobility Drills

For several reasons, older people should perform mobility drills when starting a workout program. First, these drills help to increase the range of motion, flexibility, balance, and coordination. As we age, these are often areas of decline, and injury is more likely if these areas are not addressed. Mobility and stability drills help to re-establish strength, mobility, and coordination. Also, mobility drills are necessary for a safe and effective workout program, especially for elderly populations. They improve proprioception, balance, and range of motion, all of which can help to reduce the risk of falls and injuries. Additionally, improved mobility can lower the risk of stroke by increasing the oxygen supply to the brain and improving muscle strength, which can help prevent clogged arteries

Do Proper Warm-ups and Cool Downs

It's always best to do proper warm-ups and cool-downs when starting a regular exercise routine, as it can help to reduce the risk of injury, which may be more likely to occur as we age. A proper warm-up should involve engaging the major muscle groups through stretching and dynamic movements to increase circulation and elevate the body temperature. Following a workout, a cool-down can help in aiding the return of the body to a resting state. The cool-down should also include stretching the major muscle groups to reduce any risk of the muscles becoming stiff and sore following a workout. Cooling down also helps the body gradually return to a rested state and prevents any immediate changes in posture or movement which could lead to injury. This can be especially beneficial for older adults who may have already been suffering from pre-existing medical conditions and injuries, which could be made worse with a lack of cooling down following exercise. In conclusion, proper warm-ups and cool-downs should be part of every regular elderly exercise routine in order to reduce the risk of injury and help the body return to a resting state.

Progress Slowly Over Time

Progressive overload is a technique used to increase the difficulty and intensity of exercise over time gradually. The idea is to push the body beyond its usual capabilities so that it is forced to adapt and become stronger. It would be best to take it slowly when starting an exercise routine to avoid any possible risks of injury or burnout. Perform the same routine on alternate days for at least one month before making increases in complexity. It is important to gradually increase the complexity of exercises and gradually increase the weight, repetition, and intensity of movement if you are physically able. This will allow for a steady progression and more effective health, strength, and overall fitness gains.

Know Your Limits

Seniors should know their limits when starting an exercise program because they may have age-related conditions or physical limitations that can cause them to overexert themselves. This can lead to fatigue, dehydration, injuries, and other complications. It is essential that seniors begin an exercise program with lower-impact activities such as stretching, walking, or swimming to build up strength, endurance, and balance before attempting higher-impact activities. Knowing their physical limits will also help seniors determine appropriate exercise goals and ensure they exercise safely.

CONCLUSION

Regardless of age, getting in shape and staying that way through a structured workout regimen can be daunting and intimidating. But with the proper guidance and support, committing to a regular exercise regimen can bring many rewards for improved emotional, mental, and physical health and well-being. By taking the necessary steps and arming yourself with the proper knowledge and resources, you can confidently step out of FEAR and into FREEDOM, making your exercise fitness journey a healthy and enjoyable part of your life. In doing so, you'll be significantly improving the quality of your life and putting yourself on the path to a healthier and happier future.

5

MOBILITY

The importance of enhancing mobility for seniors aged 60 and older cannot be overstated. Although seniors tend to have more limited mobility due to age-related wear and tear, investing in a good mobility plan is essential for preserving their physical health and well-being. Mobility is a significant factor in determining how physically active an older adult can be, and regular physical activity is linked to many important health benefits. In this chapter, I will share how mobility can affect older adults, the benefits of keeping up physical fitness, and the various strategies seniors can use to maximize their mobility. I will discuss the importance of being mindful of safety considerations when designing an exercise program tailored to the needs of seniors. By understanding the importance of mobility and how to maintain it, you will have the tools you need to stay healthy, active, and independent into your later years.

WHAT IS MOBILITY?

Mobility is the ability of a joint or body part to move freely and actively within a given area. A limb can move around an axis of rotation. For example, when you raise your arm over your head, the shoulder joint is responsible for the arm's mobility in this movement, allowing it to rotate around the shoulder joint. Mobility and range of motion are essential not only for older adults but for people of all ages. Increasing mobility and range of motion enables better posture, which can help reduce pain and fatigue. Additionally, it aids in joint protection, reducing the risk of injury. Furthermore, having a wide range of motion leads to increased balance and coordination, as well as better overall performance in all activities such as walking, bending, lifting, playing sports, and exercise. Finally, having greater mobility and range of motion can help with mental health and well-being, as increased mobility can help reduce stress and improve sleep.

Working on one's mobility helps decrease the likelihood of injuries by improving range of motion and flexibility, which allows the body to move more efficiently, thus reducing the risk of joint, tissue, and muscle strain associated with movement. Increased mobility also helps decrease the likelihood of injury by allowing the body to move with greater control, coordination, and stability. Aside from that, increased mobility encourages better posture, which can reduce the risk of developing chronic and long-term joint pain. Working on mobility also aids in increasing strength, balance, and stability, which all minimize the risk of injury, especially when engaging in physical activity or sport. Finally, working on your mobility will help you adapt to different movements more effectively, which reduces the risk of overuse injuries and acute traumas.

Mobility vs. Flexibility

Mobility and flexibility are closely related to physical qualities but differ. Mobility is the ability to move a joint through a full range of motion using a combination of muscle strength, joint stability, and control. Flexibility is the ability to stretch a muscle or joint as far as it can go without causing injury. Mobility is more concerned with proper joint movement and control and is essential for performing exercises safely. Flexibility is more focused on muscle tissue relaxation and elongation, which can lead to improved joint range of motion when appropriately stretched. Mobility allows for the optimization of function and performance, while flexibility increases muscle and joint health. Mobility and flexibility are vital in order to maintain a healthy body.

Flexibility is typically achieved through prolonged muscle stretches that are designed to elongate muscle fibers over time through practice. Mobility is better achieved through perfectly executed movements that promote a full range of motion across various joints. Dynamic exercises are typically more effective than stretching for improving mobility because they actively engage several muscles and joints in complex movement patterns, while stretching focuses primarily on lengthening a muscle. It promotes a more significant amount of coordination and control of movement. Increased coordination and control encourage better motor learning, leading to improved mobility.

Additionally, dynamic exercises often require the use of core muscles to help stabilize the body during movement, whereas stretching is usually done without core engagement. Dynamic exercises help to strengthen the core and can improve overall mobility. In addition to being more effective for improving mobility, dynamic movements such as heel-toe-walk, high knees, arm circles, and hip circles are also better for preventing injuries as they can strengthen the muscles, ligaments, and tendons around the joints, which can help to support them and reduce the risk of injury. That is why your Warm-Up and Cool Down sessions are essential.

THE IMPORTANCE OF BODY MOBILITY FOR SENIORS

I've talked a lot about mobility and how it differs from flexibility. But what does that mean for you as a person who identifies as a senior? A few reasons why you should dedicate more time and effort to improving your mobility will be discussed below.

Increase Muscle Mass and Strength

Improving mobility can help you increase muscle mass and strength in several ways. First, mobility exercises involve dynamic movements, which can activate muscles and provide resistance in both the concentric and eccentric phases of the movement. It can help build muscle, as it encourages muscles to contract against resistance. It also facilitates improved motor coordination and balance. Second, improving mobility helps prevent the stiffening of joints, which can lead to a reduced range of motion (ROM). Increased ROM allows for better muscle contraction, which can then lead to increased muscle mass and strength. Finally, improving mobility can also help reduce the risk of injury. When muscles and joints are stiff, your body is not able to move the way it should, leading to an increased risk of joint and muscle damage.

Greater Confidence

Mobility helps you maintain your independence. Improved mobility can allow you to move around with confidence and less fear of injury, which offers a degree of autonomy and freedom that may be lacking if your mobility is limited. It can also help ease the transition into aging, as being able to move with relative freedom can bring some confidence, control, and stability in an otherwise uncertain stage. Improving your mobility can also reduce the risk of falls, which is particularly important as older adults tend to be at an increased risk of falling. Finally, improved mobility can alleviate the feeling of being a burden on others, as someone with limited finance and mobility may rely heavily on family or friends for transportation or errands. All of these benefits can provide you with a greater sense of confidence, peace of mind, and independence.

Better Quality of Life

Better mobility can help you stay engaged with your community, family, friends, and daily activities by providing you with increased access to necessary services, transportation, and social opportunities. For example, having access to reliable transportation can help you stay connected to friends and family, attend events, and access medical care necessary for a higher quality of life. Additionally, improved mobility can reduce the risk of injury by providing you with safer alternatives, such as walk-in showers and stair-lifts, or by helping you stay active and physically fit through the use of mobility aids and technology. Improved access to physical activity can help you maintain strength, flexibility, and balance, which are beneficial for overall physical, mental, and emotional health. Finally, better mobility can provide a sense of independence and freedom for seniors, which can help them feel more connected to their environment and less isolated.

Improved Brain Function

Having improved mobility can help you improve cognitive function in many ways. First, physical activity, including exercise, is known to help improve cognitive function – in individuals of all ages. Improved mobility means you have the ability to get out and engage in physical activity, which can have many mental health benefits beyond improving cognitive function. Furthermore, enhanced mobility allows you to remain socially active, as you are more likely to be able to get out and visit with others or engage in activities in the community. This socialization helps to keep the mind active and challenged, leading to improved cognitive function.

Additionally, good mobility is necessary for proper nutrition—improved mobility makes grocery shopping and the preparation of meals easier. Eating a healthy diet of nutritious foods is known to improve cognitive function. Finally, maintaining good mobility helps you safely perform tasks around the home, keep up with necessary housework and errands, and remain independent for longer, all of which can reduce stress and lead to improved cognitive function.

Prevent or Delay Falls, Diabetes, and Strokes

Lastly, you are just a lot healthier when you make an effort to improve your mobility. First, by improving balance, flexibility, and coordination, you can reduce and prevent accidental falls, which pose the most significant risk for injury and hospitalization, as I've already mentioned. Particular muscle and joint strengthening exercises can help to reduce joint pain, stiffness, and inflammation that can lead to falls. Additionally, strengthening the lower body and core muscles can help you to maintain and improve your existing mobility by challenging your physical capacity.

Aside from that, increasing physical activity has been shown to have a significant impact on the prevention of chronic conditions such as diabetes and stroke. For instance, regular movement can help to keep the body's insulin levels more stable, reducing the risk of diabetes. Additionally, improved mobility can lower the risk of stroke by increasing the supply of oxygen to the brain and improving muscle strength, which can help prevent clogged arteries.

IMPROVING MOBILITY

When it comes to improving mobility and range of motion in a human being, there will always be some variance in terms of which parts of the body certain people will require more focus. However, as it relates to older adults, here are the areas wherein mobility improvement should be prioritized:

- neck
- shoulders
- upper arms
- hips
- hamstrings
- quadriceps
- ankles

There are many different exercises that are fully designed to help improve your range of motion and overall mobility. However, there's no need to overcomplicate the process either. Of course, it should go without saying that you should always consult the expertise of licensed physicians before embarking on any kind of exercise routine. But for the most part, there are specific exercises that are incredibly safe and effective at helping keep muscles limber and active. This can include activities like walking, yoga, dancing, swimming, cycling, and even light jogging. Any kind of exercise that promotes safe and holistic movement can help keep muscles limber and prevent them from getting stiff over time is beneficial.

Some of the best mobility exercises that are designed to help keep your vital muscles and joints as healthy and as supple as possible while you age are discussed below.

Upper Body Clam Shell

The upper body clam shell exercise is an effective movement that helps strengthen, balance, and stabilize the muscles to improve your mobility. This exercise increases the range of motion in the hips and core muscles, which can help reduce back pain, improve posture, and increase flexibility. Additionally, it can help with balance and coordination by strengthening the muscles that support the hips and lower back, which can help prevent falls.

When performing the upper body clam shell exercise, it is essential to maintain proper form and keep the core engaged and the spine straight.

The steps to perform the upper body clam shell exercise safely are as follows:

1. Begin by lying on your side with your hips, knees, and ankles stacked. Place your hands behind your head, or place one hand on the ground for stability.
2. Engage your core muscles and lift your upper body off the ground.

3. Slowly raise your top leg towards the ceiling while ensuring that your core stays engaged and your lower body is stable.
4. Hold this position for a few seconds, then lower your top leg back down without allowing your lower back to sag.
5. Repeat this exercise 8-10 times on each side for a complete set.

Semi-Sits

The semi-sits exercise is an exercise specifically designed for older adults. It is also intended to increase the range of motion in the hips and provide better mobility. It is especially beneficial for those with limited mobility due to age-related conditions such as arthritis or joint pain.

The steps on how to perform the semi-sits exercise safely include:

1. Begin standing with your feet hip-distance apart.
2. Bend your knees slightly, then slowly lower yourself into a semi-sitting position with your thighs parallel to the ground and your hands resting at your sides.
3. Hold this position for a few seconds before slowly returning to the standing position. If your balance is a concern, perform these with your back against the wall.
4. Perform this exercise for eight reps for two sets, pausing for a few seconds between each rep.

Seated Abdominal Press

The seated abdominal press is an exercise designed to target your abdominal muscles, improve core strength, and aid in flexibility, balance, and coordination. This exercise is beneficial for you, as it helps to improve mobility and reduce the risk of falling. The seated abdominal press can also help older adults build strength in their core muscles, making them less susceptible to injuries and improving posture.

To perform the seated abdominal press safely, follow these steps:

1. Sit up straight in a chair with your feet flat on the floor, approximately hip-width apart.
2. Place your hands on your thighs, palms facing up.
3. Inhale, and as you exhale, press your hands down against your thighs as firmly as you can and draw your navel in toward your spine as you hold for 10-15 seconds.
4. Slowly release the pressure on your thighs and repeat the exercise for 10-15 repetitions.

It is vital only to perform the number of repetitions that cause slight muscular fatigue in the abdominal muscles; stop once you feel any sharp pain or discomfort. Additionally, avoid any sudden or jerky movements.

Side Bends

The side bends exercise is a simple and effective exercise that helps to improve flexibility, increase mobility, and strengthen the core muscles of seniors. It targets the abdominal and lower back muscles, as well as the obliques and hips. The exercise also helps to promote balance and build stability in the core, improving overall posture.

To perform the side bends exercise safely, follow these steps:

1. Stand with your feet slightly wider than shoulder-width apart, with your toes pointing forward. Sit if standing or maintaining balance is a concern.
2. Bend at your hips and knees to lower your body, keeping your back and core straight and your head in line with your spine.
3. Place your hands on your hips and, holding your core tight, slowly lean to the left side and then back to the center.
4. Then, lean to the right side and then back to the center.
5. Repeat 10-15 times on each side.

Low-Back Rotation Stretch

The low-back rotation stretch is an exercise that helps improve your mobility by loosening up tight muscles in the lower back. This exercise is performed by lying flat on your back on the floor or on a firm bed, then crossing one leg over the opposite knee. The hands should then be placed behind the thigh, and your top knee should be gently pulled towards the chest to stretch the muscles across the lower back. This exercise is beneficial to older adults because it can help improve their range of motion and reduce any stiffness caused by inactivity.

When performing this exercise, it is wise to take it slow and not overstretch.

1. Begin by lying on a comfortable, flat surface such as a bed, yoga mat, or rug.
2. Cross one leg over the other and place the hands behind the thigh to keep the stretch in place.
3. Slowly pull the knee towards the chest until a gentle stretch is felt.
4. Hold a few seconds before gently releasing the stretch and repeating the exercise on the other side.

It is essential to be mindful of pain and discomfort during this exercise. If any pain or discomfort is felt, stopping and discussing the activity with a doctor before continuing is recommended. When done correctly and on a regular basis, the low back rotation stretch can help improve your mobility and can provide many benefits for overall health and well-being.

CONCLUSION

In conclusion, mobility exercises are an essential part of your fitness routine. These exercises can increase strength, flexibility, balance, and overall health. They can help to reduce the risk of falls, improve physical endurance, and even help to relieve joint pain. Additionally, these exercises can increase your physical and mental well-being by providing a sense of accomplishment, improving mood, and helping to reduce stress. Although these exercises may seem daunting initially, you can gradually build upon their abilities with patience and consistency. Mobility exercises are an excellent way to take control of aging by staying physically active and mobile for many years to come.

6

THE MIND-MUSCLE CONNECTION

"One day you are going to look back and see how far you have come."

— BIANCA APARACINO

Welcome to the world of mind-muscle connections! In this chapter, you will learn a bit about what the mind-muscle connection is, why it is essential, and the best practices for developing, strengthening, and maintaining these connections over time.

The mind-muscle connection is an important concept in the world of human performance. It refers to the link between the mind and the muscles of the body and how they work together to create optimal performance. The strength of this connection affects our ability to move, respond, and perform at our best during workouts and sports activities.

Unfortunately, many myths have been floated around about the mind-muscle connection. To start with, there is a belief that developing a powerful mind-muscle connection makes us stronger and faster seemingly overnight. This is not true. The concept of the mind-muscle connection has been around for centuries, and it is still the same today. Developing a powerful mind-muscle connection requires time, dedication, and practice.

In the upcoming sections, I will discuss more specific ways to practice and strengthen this connection. However, it is important to note that the process of developing a strong mind-muscle connection requires patience, hard work, and consistency. Achieving optimal performance does not happen overnight, and keeping a solid mind-muscle relationship takes ongoing practice over time.

By the end of this chapter, you will understand the mind-muscle connection and the best ways to practice and strengthen it. You will learn about common myths related to the mind-muscle connection, the importance of practice and consistency in developing mind-muscle connections, and the best practices for strengthening these connections over time.

Let's get started!

UNDERSTANDING THE MIND-MUSCLE CONNECTION

The mind-muscle connection is a phenomenon in which the mind contracts and focuses on individual muscles rather than simply moving a limb. This is often done in order to maximize muscular force or to increase the efficiency of a specific exercise. It is often seen as the missing link between performing an effective workout and simply going through the motions.

When you think about it, the mind-muscle connection isn't anything new. In the past, many athletes, bodybuilders, and lifters have understood and practiced this concept, often in pursuit of muscle gain and strength. Their ability to focus on specific muscles during training has allowed them to dominate their goals. However, in recent years, it has blown up as a 'trend' among fitness enthusiasts.

At its core, the mind-muscle connection is simply a technique that involves focusing on the muscles during a given exercise rather than just the activity itself. This technique has been found to increase the intensity and activation of the desired muscle group and, thus, help you target it more directly.

Practically speaking, the best way to create the mind-muscle connection is to mentally create tension in the working muscle group while actively engaging it. For instance, when doing a chest press, you should imagine your chest muscles contracting and consciously attempting to squeeze them during each repetition. This same concept can be applied to any muscle group in any exercise, making it an excellent focus technique for those looking to increase intensity and results in the gym. It is vital to complete the repetitions in a slow and controlled manner. Doing this will allow you to pay closer attention to the contraction and relaxation of the muscle.

The mind-muscle connection isn't an instant fix to achieving the fitness level or body form you want; it takes time and practice to master. However, it is definitely an effective technique to help you target muscles more efficiently and effectively. As such, if you're looking to make the most of your exercises, then the mind-muscle connection is worth keeping in mind.

In order for the mind-muscle connection to be effective, you need to be aware of the muscles they are working and take the time to focus on your actions. A simple example is a bicep curl. When you are performing this exercise, you should focus on the contraction of your bicep and make sure that the muscles are engaging properly. Creating tension in specific muscle groups in your body will enable you to gain strength in all the right areas, legs, back, abs, etc. This will help you get the most out of the exercise and create a stronger connection between the mind and muscles.

Apart from just focusing on the exercise itself, it is also important to use visualization techniques to enhance the effectiveness of your workout further. Visualization techniques help to better connect to the muscles and visualize the specific movements they need to perform. For example, when performing a bicep curl, take your time to envision the bicep muscle pulling your arm towards your shoulder and then contracting and releasing as you perform the exercise. This visualization type will help recruit all of the muscle fibers necessary to complete the activity effectively.

By having a more intentional awareness and clarity while exercising, you will be able to improve the quality and efficiency of your movements as well as build strength and rehabilitation progress over time. The mind-muscle connection is vital for seniors who want to improve balance, mobility, and strength for life.

MIND-MUSCLE CONNECTION MYTHS

The myths surrounding the mind-muscle connection have been around for centuries and have recently proven to affect how people approach their mental and physical health profoundly. In this section, we will take a closer look at these myths and why it's particularly important for seniors to be aware of them when developing an exercise routine. With this new knowledge in hand, seniors can create an exercise routine that is both safe and beneficial to their overall health and well-being.

Myth: Mind-Muscle Connection Works the Same for Everyone

The myth that the mind-muscle connection works the same for everyone is based on the assumption that all individuals are capable of achieving the same level and intensity of muscle contraction when activating a specific muscle group. In reality, this is not the case. While everyone has the potential to learn how to start a particular muscle through mind-muscle connection, the level of engagement and the capability of achieving intense contractions vary significantly among individuals. Factors such as muscle type, body composition, personal history, experience, and genetics can all impact the degree to which an individual can contract a specific muscle. As such, it is essential to tailor your mind-muscle connection exercises to account for your physical characteristics and personal goals.

Myth: Beginners Should Always Focus on Mind-Muscle Connection

The myth that beginners should always focus on mind-muscle connection is based on the belief that by concentrating on the relationship between your mind and a particular muscle group, you can amplify the effects of your exercise and potentially increase overall muscular growth. Practicing this enables you to create a stronger mind-muscle connection that can help you perform and control the movement of the target muscle group more effectively, requiring less effort and resulting in more contraction. This can help to build strength and size faster and encourage your mind to be more aware of the area you are working in. While this has benefits and can be a helpful exercise tool, it should not be the only focus of a beginner's routine. Beginners still need to ensure that their workout plan is well-balanced and varied, with adequate rest and recovery time and the proper time for form and technique development.

Myth: Mind-Muscle Connection Gives You Instant Strength

This myth suggests that when a person focuses their entire mind on a particular movement or muscle group, they can instantly 'will' themselves to lift more weight or move more efficiently than they could have before. Essentially, the idea is that if a person can visualize the exact movements they need to make, they will be able to increase strength and power in that specific muscle group.

The truth is, while the mind-muscle connection can certainly increase performance and efficiency, it won't give one instant strength. It takes weeks, months, and sometimes years of practice and hard work for one to build muscle and power over time. Additionally, the mind-muscle connection should be viewed as something other than a replacement for proper technique and form when it comes to lifting or performing any exercise. Mind-muscle connection should be used in conjunction with appropriate technique and form for one to become stronger, faster, and more powerful.

Myth: Mind Muscle Connection Works All the Time for Every Exercise

The myth that the mind-muscle connection works all the time for every exercise suggests that by simply focusing your thoughts on a particular muscle group during motion, you can engage it more intensely and, therefore, achieve better results and faster gains. While it is true that focusing on the intended muscle group and engaging it entirely through the proper form can lead to better results, the idea that this will happen all the time with every exercise needs to be more accurate. Additionally, activities vary in difficulty and complexity, which can affect how much mind-muscle connection can be achieved. Furthermore, some people find it difficult to establish a mind-muscle connection because they cannot mentally focus on the target muscle group throughout the duration of the exercise. This is why it is important to consistently exercise and focus on form, breathing, and body position when exercising to ensure proper engagement of the intended muscle group.

HOW TO DEVELOP THE MIND-MUSCLE CONNECTION

Developing a strong mind-muscle connection is essential for strengthening and toning muscles, increasing the range of motion, improving coordination, and preventing injuries. This section will explain how to develop the mind-muscle connection while considering an older adult's particular needs.

Warm Up for Every Exercise

Warming up before every exercise helps to build your mind-muscle connection by adequately preparing the body for exercise. Aside from that, warming up helps to increase blood flow to the working muscles, which can reduce the risk of injury and make the muscles suppler and ready for the activity. Warm-ups can also help you get their minds into the right state for a workout by assisting them to focus on the action and increase their level of awareness. Warming up can help create a better connection between their muscles and the mind, which can be beneficial for you in a variety of different exercises and activities.

Lift Light

Lifting lighter weights can help build the mind-muscle connection by allowing you to focus on the form of the exercise and the movement of the muscle. With light weights, you can more easily focus on the subtleties of the action, such as engaging the muscles at the correct points of the exercise; this will allow you to create a stronger connection between your mind and the working muscle. This connection can improve brain function, as it helps link movement and thoughts together, as well as increase strength and progression. As you progress and become stronger, you can begin to add more weight to increase the challenge of the exercise.

Move Slowly

Moving slowly during workouts can help you build your mind-muscle connection in several ways:

1. You can focus on the targeted muscles more intensely by slowing down the movements. The process of slowing down will ensure that the right muscles are being activated and engaged throughout the exercise.
2. By taking the time to move slowly, allows you to better focus on proper form and alignment. This will help ensure that your movements are done correctly and safely, decreasing their risk of injury.
3. Moving slowly allows you to practice focusing on the task at hand and staying present during the workout, which is beneficial for any age.
4. By maintaining the same slow pace throughout the workout, you can build up their endurance so that they can eventually increase the speed of the movements.

Flex Between Sets

Flexing between sets can help you build your mind-muscle connection by activating the nerves and muscle fibers associated with a particular exercise. This practice can increase the body's awareness of the movement, engage more muscle fibers, and increase the intensity of the activity. Building a strong mind-muscle connection may lead to better movement control and increased muscle activation, both of which can help to make the most of their workout. Performing flexing exercises between sets can also introduce opportunities for balance and coordination drills and help improve muscular endurance.

CONCLUSION

Overall, the mind-muscle connection is a powerful concept when it comes to exercise that anyone can apply. In particular, for older adults who are just beginning their workout routine, the mind-muscle connection is a great way to ensure that each movement is done correctly and with proper form to maximize the benefits of their workouts and stay injury-free. Additionally, keeping a clear head and becoming aware of each muscle can help them gain a better awareness of their body and what it is capable of. While proper form and technique should always be a priority, using the mind-muscle connection can help ensure that the movements are being done purposefully. Therefore, it is an invaluable tool that can be used to enhance any workout routine.

7

THE AGING PROCESS – A FACT OF LIFE

As we age, our bodies go through a variety of changes that can often be difficult to accept. It can be an unsettling feeling! I know. No one wants to entertain thoughts of their own personal body deterioration over time. However, it's important to note that aging is a natural part of life, and it can bring a variety of emotional, physical, and mental changes. From wrinkles and gray hair to aching joints and declining muscle mass, the aging process can be a difficult journey. However, there are ways to successfully cope with these changes that come along with aging. In this chapter, I will explore the aging process, its accompanying changes, and how to cope with them. I will share the various ways our bodies change as we age, from the appearance of wrinkles to the decline in muscle mass and bone density. This chapter will give you a more profound and holistic perspective on aging and help you understand how your body changes over time.

One positive fact about aging is that the average life expectancy has increased significantly over the last century. In 1900, the average life expectancy was just 47 years old. Today, the average life expectancy is 78 years of age. This increase is due to advances in medicine and healthcare, as well as improved nutrition and healthier lifestyle choices. Additionally, you might need to be aware that the risk of developing certain diseases increases with age. For example, the risk of developing Alzheimer's disease doubles every five years after age 65. By age 85, the risk of developing Alzheimer's is nearly 30%. Maintaining a consistent exercise routine will add great value to lowering this risk.

Another side effect of aging is that your body can become less efficient as years pass. There is difficulty in regulating body temperature, maintaining muscle mass, and healing from injuries. This state can make it difficult for you to stay active and healthy. These are just a few of the interesting facts about the aging process. While aging is a natural process, it's important to be aware of the potential risks associated with it. By understanding the facts about aging, you can make informed decisions about your health and well-being. Ultimately, aging is inevitable, but that doesn't mean it's beyond our control. You still have the power to make good choices that will help you to live a long, strong, and healthy life moving forward. Aging may be inevitable, but healthy, graceful aging should be your reality!

WHY DO WE AGE?

Simply put, we all age because time is relentless, and life has an expiration date. As we age, we are reminded of our mortality and the fragility of life. The passing of time brings with it a sense of loss and regret as we reflect on the years that have gone by and the opportunities that have passed us by. It can be a difficult and emotional journey, but it is ultimately a necessary one, as getting old is an unavoidable part of life.

Aging is a process that should be embraced, not feared. It is a natural part of life that brings with it a wealth of wisdom and experience that can be shared with others. Aging doesn't always have to mean physical decline. Maintaining a healthy lifestyle and eating a balanced diet can help. There are different types of aging that can be experienced, such as emotional, spiritual, and mental growth.

Aging can be a powerful motivator. It can bring a newfound appreciation for life and an increased ability to be present at the moment. It can also develop a deeper understanding of oneself and the world around us. Embracing aging can be a beautiful journey of self-discovery that should be celebrated.

Types of Aging

Cellular Aging

Cellular aging is the process by which cells in the body become less efficient over time and eventually stop functioning. It is a natural part of the aging process, resulting from a combination of factors, including genetic, environmental, lifestyle choices, etc.

At the cellular level, aging is characterized by a decrease in healthy cells and an increase in damaged or mutated cells within your body. As cells age, their ability to function decreases. They become less able to divide and replicate, leading to a decrease in their ability to regenerate and repair themselves. The mitochondria, the powerhouses of the cell, become less efficient and produce fewer energy molecules, leading to a decrease in the amount of energy available for the cell to use. Additionally, cells produce less of the proteins and enzymes necessary for normal cellular processes, leading to a decrease in the ability of the cell to carry out its normal functions.

Finally, as cells age, their DNA becomes more damaged and mutated, increasing genetic mutations. These mutations can lead to a variety of health problems, including cancer, heart disease, and other age-related diseases. As a result, cells become more susceptible to damage from environmental toxins, UV radiation, and other sources.

Damage-Related and Environmental Aging

Damage-related aging is the process of physical, chemical, and biological changes that occur in an organism over time due to damage from external sources. Various sources, including ultraviolet radiation, toxic chemicals, and environmental stressors, can cause this exposure. Damage-related aging can lead to multiple health problems, such as wrinkles, age spots, and age-related diseases.

On the other hand, environmental aging is the process of physical, chemical, and biological changes that occur in an organism over time due to environmental factors. This includes changes due to pollution, climate change, and other environmental stressors. Environmental aging can lead to various health issues like respiratory diseases, cancer, and cardiovascular diseases. This also causes changes in the physical appearance of an organism.

Both kinds of aging are closely related and are often closely linked with one another. Whatever the case, when your body has been exposed to specific stressors and environmental factors, there is a good chance that cellular changes will occur due to that exposure.

Why Do Life Expectancies Increase?

Life expectancies increase over time due to healthcare, nutrition, and lifestyle improvements. The more active you are, the better. Advances in medical technology have allowed for earlier detection and treatment of diseases, leading to a decrease in mortality rates. Additionally, better sanitation and improved nutrition have allowed people to live longer, stronger, healthier lives. Furthermore, lifestyle changes such as quitting smoking, exercising regularly, and eating a balanced diet have all contributed to increasing quality of life and expiration. Lastly, increased access to healthcare, including preventive care, has helped to reduce mortality rates and increase life expectancies.

Why Do Women Live Longer Than Men?

Women generally live longer than men because of biological and lifestyle factors. From a biological perspective, women tend to have a more robust immune system than men, which helps them fight off illnesses and diseases more effectively. Additionally, women have a higher level of estrogen, which helps protect their heart health and reduce the risk of cardio-vascular disease. From a lifestyle perspective, women are like-lier to take better care of themselves than men. Women are more likely to go to the doctor for regular checkups, and they are more likely to follow their doctor's advice. Women are also more likely to maintain a healthy diet and exercise regularly, which can help reduce their risk of chronic diseases. Overall, these biological and lifestyle factors contribute to women living longer than men.

Can We Slow Down the Effects of Aging?

The effects of aging can be slowed down in several ways, but one of the most important is to live a healthier lifestyle. Staying active means engaging in physical activity, such as walking, running, biking, swimming, or any other form of exercise that gets your heart pumping and your muscles moving. Not only does physical activity help keep your body strong and healthy, but it can also help keep your mind sharp and alert.

In addition to physical activity, there are other ways to slow down the effects of aging. Eating a healthy diet with plenty of organic fruits, vegetables, incorporating blends of fruit and vegetable juices, and whole grains can help to reduce inflammation, which is one of the critical factors in the aging process. Eating foods rich in antioxidants can also help protect your cells from damage caused by free radicals, which can accelerate the aging process. It is also essential to get plenty of sleep. Sleep helps to repair and rejuvenate the body, and it can help to reduce stress and improve your overall well-being. Aim for 7-8 hours of sleep each night, and make sure to get to bed at a reasonable hour of the day or night.

Lastly, it is important to stay socially active. You will be maintaining consistent communication with your circle. Join local community organizations. Socializing and engaging in meaningful activities can keep your mind sharp, reduce stress, and improve overall well-being. Aside from that, staying social is also an effective way to exercise your mental, spiritual, and emotional acuities. By following these tips, you are giving yourself the best shot at slowing down the effects of aging and staying healthy and active for many decades.

THE STAGES OF AGING

Aging is a personal process and journey that everyone goes through. Each of these journeys is unique and special to every individual. That's why one person's aging process isn't necessarily going to look exactly like another person's. Having said that, there are still some general stages of aging that people go through at different points of their life: Self-Sufficiency, Interdependence, Dependence, Crisis Management, and End of Life.

Self-Sufficiency in Your 60s)

The self-sufficiency stage of aging is the period of life in which an individual can take care of their own needs and manage their own life. During this stage, individuals can make decisions for themselves, manage their finances, and take care of their health and safety. They may also be able to work and be involved in social activities.

This aging stage is important as it allows individuals to remain independent and in control of their own lives. It can also be a time of great satisfaction, as individuals can take pride in their accomplishments and enjoy the fruits of their labor. However, it is important to note that some individuals may still require assistance during this stage, and it is crucial to ensure they receive the necessary support.

Interdependence (70s and 80s)

The interdependence stage of aging is a period of life in which some individuals can no longer live independently and must rely on others for assistance with activities of daily living and instrumental activities of daily living. This aging stage characterizes decreased physical and cognitive abilities and increased reliance on others for help. The interdependence stage can be caused by a variety of factors, including age-related illnesses, physical disabilities, mental health issues, and cognitive decline. During this stage, some individuals may need assistance with tasks such as bathing, dressing, and eating, as well as more complex tasks such as managing finances, shopping, and transportation. This stage of aging can be difficult for both the individual and the caregivers, as the individual may feel a sense of loss of independence and autonomy. In addition, the caregiver may experience stress, fatigue, and a sense of responsibility. It is important to ensure that individuals in the interdependency stage are provided with the necessary support and resources to ensure that they can live as independently as possible.

Dependence (80+)

The dependence stage of aging refers to the period of life when an individual can no longer take care of themselves and needs assistance from others to maintain their health and well-being. This aging stage is often characterized by physical decline, cognitive decline, and increased reliance on others for care. During this stage, most individuals may experience a range of changes such as decreased mobility, difficulty with daily activities, and increased risk of falls and fractures.

At this stage, individuals may need assistance with activities of daily living such as bathing, dressing, and eating. They may also need help with managing their medications and other medical tasks. Family members and caretakers must provide support and assistance with these tasks to ensure that the individual's needs are met. Additionally, providing social support and companionship can help to reduce feelings of loneliness and isolation.

It is important to note that the dependence stage of aging is not an inevitable part of aging and is not necessarily a negative experience. With the proper support, individuals can remain independent and active for as long as possible.

Crisis Management

This stage of aging is a period of time when an individual is faced with the need to manage a crisis or a significant life event. This stage is characterized by a heightened sense of vulnerability and a need to cope with the changes that come with aging.

The crisis management stage can include various events such as illness, death of a loved one, retirement, and other major changes. During this stage, individuals may experience multiple emotions, such as fear, anxiety, anger, and sadness. They may also experience physical changes such as fatigue, decreased mobility, and decreased ability to perform daily tasks.

At this stage, individuals may need help from family, friends, and professionals to manage the changes and cope with the emotions they are experiencing. They may also need to make decisions about their future, such as whether to move to a retirement home or stay there.

The crisis management stage of aging can be challenging, but it is a part of the aging process. It can be a time of growth, learning, and self-discovery as individuals come to terms with their changing circumstances and develop new skills to cope with them. With the proper support, this stage can be a time of growth and transformation.

CHANGES IN THE BODY WITH AGING

As was discussed, your body goes through many different changes as it ages over time. We all do. The difference is in the way these changes occur. Here are some more specific details on the changes in your body as you age. Remember that there are preventative measures you can employ right now to live healthier. A consistent fitness and nutritional program can add tremendous value to your life as you age. If you need assistance, join my team.

Cardiovascular System

The cardiovascular system changes as a result of aging in several ways. The heart's ability to pump blood decreases, decreasing the amount of oxygen and nutrients delivered to the body's organs and tissues. The walls of the arteries become thicker and stiffer, making them less able to expand and contract with each heartbeat. As a result, the heart has to work harder to pump blood throughout the body. The heart's valves also become less efficient, decreasing the amount of blood that can be pumped. Finally, the veins become less elastic, which can reduce the amount of blood returning to the heart. These changes can lead to an increased risk of heart disease and stroke.

Bones, Joints, and Muscles

Our bones, joints, and muscles all experience changes as we age. Bones become more brittle and less dense due to decreased calcium and other minerals in the body. Joints may become stiffer and less flexible due to a decrease in cartilage and synovial fluid, as well as an increase in bone spurs. Muscles may become weaker due to the decline in muscle mass and a reduction in the body's ability to repair muscle fibers. These changes can lead to an increased risk of falls and other injuries.

Digestive System

As we age, the digestive system becomes less efficient due to decreased digestive enzymes, gastric acid, and bile production. The muscles in the digestive tract become weaker, leading to slower digestion and emptying of the stomach. The small intestine becomes less able to absorb nutrients, resulting in poor nutrition. In addition, the salivary glands produce less saliva, leading to a dry mouth and difficulty swallowing. The chewing also becomes slower as teeth and gums weaken with age. These factors contribute to the digestive system becoming less effective with age.

Bladder and Urinary Tract

When you age, the bladder's walls become thicker and less elastic, making it harder for the bladder to hold urine for long periods. This can lead to more frequent urination and even incontinence. The urinary tract also becomes narrower, slowing the passage of urine and making it easier for bacteria to grow and cause infections. Lastly, the muscles in the bladder may become weaker and less able to contract, making it harder to empty the bladder. Kegel and pelvic floor muscle exercises are great for helping keep the walls of the bladder more elastic as seniors age. These exercises involve squeezing and releasing the muscles around the bladder and rectum.

Memory and Cognitive Function

Our ability to store and recall information, process and retain information, and respond quickly to stimuli can all be affected when we age. Memory and cognitive function generally decline with age due to physical and physiological changes in the brain. As we age, neurons in the brain may become less efficient, leading to slower processing speed, difficulty learning new information, and decreased working memory capacity. Aside from that, aging can cause a decrease in executive functions, including the ability to make decisions, plan, and prioritize, which can also lead to difficulty in problem-solving and information processing.

Eyes and Ears

The eyes and ears are two of the senses most impacted by aging. As we age, our eyes may experience a decrease in visual acuity, and our pupils may become less responsive to light. We may also experience age-related macular degeneration and cataracts, which can further reduce our vision. Regarding hearing, the most common age-related condition is presbycusis, or hearing loss due to the natural aging process. This can cause difficulty in understanding speech, as well as a loss of range in hearing.

Skin

As a person ages, the skin's collagen and elastin production decreases, which keeps the skin looking firm, smooth, and elastic. As a result, skin loses its elasticity and becomes thinner, drier, and less able to protect itself from damage. The fatty layer below the skin also begins to thin, leading to wrinkles, age spots, and decreased skin tone. The skin's ability to repair itself begins to slow down, leading to reduced healing and increased scarring. Additionally, the sweat and oil glands in the skin become less active, leading to dryness, itchiness, and flakiness.

Weight

During the aging process, we tend to lose muscle and bone mass, which can lead to a decrease in overall body weight. This is because of decreased physical activity and metabolic rate, which can lead to reduced muscle mass, bone density, and fat stores. Additionally, hormonal changes can also contribute to weight loss as we age. All of these factors can lead to a decrease in weight as we age, although the amount lost will vary from person to person.

EXERCISE HELPS FIGHT AGING

Exercise is an essential component of staying healthy and promoting longevity. As we age, it becomes increasingly important to maintain an active lifestyle and engage in regular physical activity to guard against the effects of aging. Exercise has been shown to be beneficial in a number of ways when it comes to aging, from helping to maintain a healthy weight to improving physical strength and balance. Moreover, regular physical activity can help to reduce the risk of developing age-related diseases such as diabetes and heart disease. In this section, we will explore the various benefits of exercise on aging and how you can incorporate physical activity into your life. You must be consistent!

Building Muscle Strength

Regular exercise helps build muscle strength in aging people by stimulating the muscles to grow stronger and more efficient. When engaging in regular, moderate-intensity exercise, the muscles will respond by getting stronger and abler to handle daily activity demands. Strength training exercises, such as weightlifting, helps to increase muscle mass and strength, while aerobic exercises help to improve cardiovascular health and endurance. Both types of exercise help improve overall strength and endurance, which can help aging people stay independent and do the activities they enjoy.

Increasing Bone Density

The movement also increases bone density for aging people by increasing the activity of osteoblasts, the cells responsible for forming new bone tissue. Weight-bearing exercises, such as walking, running, and lifting weights, will help to stimulate the formation of new bone tissue, leading to an increase in bone density. This helps to reduce the risk of osteoporosis and other age-related bone diseases. Additionally, regular exercise can help to improve balance and coordination, which can help protect against falls and fractures.

Improving Cognitive Function

Physical activity can help aging people improve their cognitive function by increasing oxygen flow to the brain, which can help boost alertness and concentration. Exercise can also help people maintain a healthy weight, reducing the risk of age-related diseases such as dementia, Alzheimer's, and stroke. Additionally, exercise can help stimulate the release of chemicals in the brain, such as endorphins, which can reduce stress, improve mood, and increase cognitive functioning.

Lengthening Telomeres

Exercise has been shown to help slow the aging process by lengthening telomeres, which are the protective caps found at the ends of chromosomes that naturally shorten with age. As telomeres shorten, cells age and die more quickly, leading to accelerated aging. Research has shown that regular physical activity can help slow the shortening of telomeres, therefore slowing down the aging process. This is likely due to the physiological changes in the body in response to exercise, such as increased production of free radicals, which are beneficial for telomere maintenance. Additionally, exercise has been shown to positively affect psychological health, which can also play a role in telomere maintenance.

CONCLUSION

In conclusion, aging is an inevitable part of life, and various changes occur in the body as you age. Understanding the stages of aging is essential as they provide an overview of how the body and mind flow through this time. We may never know why we age, but steps can be taken to reduce the adverse effects of aging by maintaining a healthier and consistently active lifestyle. Exercise is a great way to stay fit and healthy and combat the physical and mental decline that sometimes comes with aging. Although aging is a part of life, you can use your knowledge to dominate aging. Ensure that you age as gracefully and healthily as possible.

CONCLUSION

You're never too old to start exercising, so don't waste more time. Get out there, take it step by step, and begin to feel the incredible improvements you'll experience in your quality of life. The most important thing for you to remember is that exercise should be fun and something you enjoy doing. Don't give up, and progress at your own pace. With consistency, dedication, and patience, you'll soon see results and enjoy the journey.

I've stressed over and over again how exercising regularly is an excellent way for you to stay fit and healthy as you age. By committing to a routine, adults who identify as seniors can continue to enjoy the benefits of physical activity, such as improved physical and mental well-being. This book has valuable tips and advice to help you get started and maintain the motivation necessary to stay in shape. The long-term benefits are many, if completed in a safe and controlled way.

I highlighted the importance of talking to a physician before beginning any exercise program. It is also essential to start slowly and gradually increasing the intensity level. Listening to your body is vital. Stop exercising, and consult your physician if feeling any unusual pain or discomfort before continuing.

Ultimately, exercising consistently can be a great way to stay well-rounded in body and mind. If you make a concerted effort to take care of your body and be active, you can continue to experience all the benefits of physical activity. You can have a successful and rewarding experience at any age with the right kind of guidance and motivation. At the end of the day, regular exercise can transform your life and extend your lifespan.

Congratulations on making it through this book! Now you're equipped with the knowledge and tools to start exercising and making positive changes in your life. Exercising will help you to increase your energy, overall health, and attitude. Regardless of your age or physical condition, following the routines outlined in this book and exercising regularly can improve your emotional, mental, and physical health. I hope this book has helped kick-start your journey towards a lifelong healthier life-style. With these workouts, you can expect positive results in strength, balance, cardiovascular health, flexibility, and overall independence—all while looking and feeling better. Exercise is not only beneficial for your health, but it's also lots of fun. Play your favorite songs, keep your motivation up, find activities you enjoy, and get active! Remember to celebrate EVERYTHING! Enjoy yourself!

ABOUT THE AUTHOR

Dr. Andrea Blake-Garrett is a talented author, educator, and entrepreneur known for her education and health and wellness work. She firmly believes that a healthy mind, body, and spirit are the keys to a fulfilling life. Her journey toward transformation began in December 2020, when she decided to take charge of her health and make significant changes in her lifestyle.

Dr. Blake-Garrett lost an incredible 100 pounds of body fat through sheer determination, consistency, and hard work. Her success inspired her to create Teamnoexcuses50, a health and wellness company that helps clients of all ages adopt healthier lifestyles. With her experience and knowledge in health and wellness, Dr. Blake-Garrett has made a significant impact on many people's lives.

Dr. Blake-Garrett is also an active social media user, with her Instagram handle, the "Notorious DRABG," gaining momentum. She uses her platform to share valuable insights on health and wellness, motivate and inspire her followers, and advocate for a healthy lifestyle.

As an author, Dr. Blake-Garrett has published five books. Her fourth book, *DOWN 100 Pounds! How I Used Positive Affirmations*

To Transform My Mind & Help Maximize My Weight Loss and Life! documents her journey toward weight loss and offers practical tips for others who want to follow in her footsteps. Her fifth book, *Life! Spice It Up! How To Transform and Heal With 5 Everyday Spices* highlights spices' medicinal properties and how they can be used to promote and maintain better health.

Overall, Dr. Andrea Blake-Garrett is a passionate and dedicated health and wellness advocate who has made it her mission to help others lead healthier, happier, and more fulfilling lives. Her transformation and success are a testament to her belief that anything is possible with the right mindset and accurate information.

REFERENCES

Al-Obaidi, S. M., Hittawi, M. S., & Singh, A. (2007). *Resistance exercise training attenuates hypertension and improves endothelium-dependent vasodilation in prehypertensive and hypertensive humans: A systematic review.* American Journal of Hypertension, 20(12), 1308–1317. https://doi:10.1038/sj.ajh. 0803609

Alvero, C., Brosky, J. A., Schimansky, J. B., Ropero, A. B., Vieira, A. E. & Bottaro, M. (2018). *Resistance training and sarcopenia: A systematic review of randomized controlled trials.* Frontiers in Physiology, 9(627). https://doi:10. 3389/fphys.2018.00627

Alzheimer's Association. (2020). *Exercise and Physical Activity: Get the Facts.* Retrieved 15 October 2020, from https://www.alz.org/alzheimers-demen tia/caregiving/exercise-physical-activity-facts

American Diabetes Association. (2021). *Type 2 Diabetes.* Retrieved from https://www.diabetes.org/diabetes/type-2

American Psychology Association. (2021). *Strength Training and Diabetes.* Retrieved from https://www.apa.org/pi/aging/programs/exercise/ strength-training-diabetes

Babbie, E., & Mouton, J. (2020). *The practice of social research.* Boston, MA: Wadsworth Cengage Learning.

Biddle, S. J. H., Liu, J., Batterham, A. M., & Sallis, J. F. (2014). *Physical activity and mental health in children and adolescents: A review of reviews.* British Journal of Sports Medicine, 48(11), 873-878.

Buckley, J. (2020). *How Strength Training Benefits Seniors.* Healthline. https:// www.healthline.com/health/physical-fitness/strength-training-exercises- for-seniors

Cancer.net. (2020). *"Risk Factors for Cancer in Elderly People".* Retrieved from https://www.cancer.net/navigating-cancer-care/prevention-and-healthy- living/prevention/risk-factors-cancer-elderly-people

Dwivedi, Y. K. et al. (2018). *Effect of strength training on physical and mental health in elderly persons: a systematic review and meta-analysis of randomized controlled trials.* BMC Geriatrics, 18(1), 1-12.

Duckworth, J. (2014). *Impact of physical activity on delivery of oxygen to tissues and cardiorespiratory fitness.* Sports Medicine. 44(3), 299-308.

Fano, E., Palma, A., Cannizzaro, G., Lo Castro, V., De Vita, F. & Calapai, G. (2014). *Effect of progressive resistance training on resting metabolic rate in elderly women.* Journal of Clinical Medicine Research, 6(7), 398-403. https://doi:10.14740/jocmr1645w

Friedenreich, C. M., Thorgeir Halls, T. Y., & Miller, A. B. (2007). *Cardiac rehabilitation: review of randomized controlled trials.* Canadian Medical Association Journal, 176(9), 1379-1385. Retrieved from https://www.cmaj.ca/content/176/9/1379

Hagerman, F.C., Hulsey, M.L., O'Brien, C., & Koehle, M.S. (2018). *Progressive resistance training intervention in frail elderly: Training principles, prescription and safety.* European Journal of Physical and Rehabilitation Medicine, 54(5), 771–778. Rertrieved from http://dx.doi.org/10.23736/S1973-9087.18.04847-2

Johannsen, D.L., Lowe, D.A., Smith, S.J., & DeMott, R. (2016). *Benefits of Resistance Training on Bone Mineral Density in Elderly Adults: A Meta-Analysis.* Osteoporosis International, 28(2), 559-567. https://doi:10.1007/s00198-016-3773-x

Kasza, J., Elley, C. R., Robinson, E., Beaglehole, R., OByrne, J., Salmond, C., & Jackson, R. (2007). *Cardiovascular disease mortality and morbidity in elderly people.* The New Zealand Medical Journal, 120(1262). https://www.ncbi.nlm.nih.gov/pmc/articles/PMC2063017/

Kane, S. & Mouradian, V. (2012). *Strength Training: What are the Benefits? Harvard Health Publishing.* Retrieved from https://www.health.harvard.edu/staying-healthy/strength-training-what-are-the-benefits

Kolokotroni, E., Strataki, A., & Gergianaki, I. (2018). *Resistance training effects among elderly: A Literature Review.* Hippokratia, 22(1), 7–12. https://doi.org/10.30978/HIPP.2018.22.1.10

Konzelmann, B., Mondor, C., Cadieux, G., Cournoyer, M., Rosa-Neto, P., Bocti, C. (2020). *"Strength and Resistance Training for Older Adults: Trajectories of Adherence and Quality of School".* Medicine & Science in Sports & Exercise; 52(7): 1547-1556.

Lage-Oliveira, J., Correia-Oliveira, C., Ramos, M., Silva, A. M., Costa, J. & Borralho, N. M. (2015). *Efficacy of resistance training in the elderly: A systematic review.* Revista Brasileira De Medicina De Familia E Comunidade, 10(29), 443-453.

Lauder, M. A. (2011). Core muscles: *Why strong core muscles give you more than a six pack.* Physical Therapy Reviews, 16(2), 175-181. https://doi:10.1179/174328811x12971394993859

Lee, C.-C., & Sivarajan, V. (2001). *Physiological effects of resistance training and bone mass.* Current Sports Medicine Reports, 1(2), 70-76. https://doi:10.1249/00133691-200800020-00014

Li, N., Zhao, R., Jin, T., Deng, J., & Yu, Y. (2019). *Effects of a 16-Week Strength Training Program in Older Adults with Type 2 Diabetes.* Journal of Diabetes Research, 2019, 1–7. https://doi.org/10.1155/2019/7940698

Lister-Sharp, D. (2020). *ATP and Exercise.* Retrieved November 4, 2020, from https://www.verywellfit.com/what-is-atp-in-exercise-3495119

Magnani, J., Laus, S., Pedutto, A., Solis, M., & De Stefano, G. (2008). *Metabolic effects of physical training in COPD patients: A systematic review.* Clinical Rehabilitation, 22(8), 653-665. Retrieved from https://journals.sagepub.com/doi/abs/10.1177/0269215508091739

McGowan, C. (2015). *Strength Training for Seniors: Benefits and Tips.* Retrieved August 25, 2020, from https://www.healthline.com/health/fitness-exercise/strength-training-for-seniors#benefits

Miller, C.E., Bezuidenhout, C., Bergstrom, J., Donath, L., Oldridge, N., Reaburn, P. (2017). *"Resistance Training for Healthy Aging: A Meta-Analysis".* Sports Medicine; 47(8): 1579-1590.

Miller, S. (2018). *What is Strength Training?* ACEfitness.org. Retrieved from https://www.acefitness.org/education-and-resources/lifestyle/blog/5099/what-is-strength-training

Miyajima, E., Griffiths, E., & Gaskin, C. (2011). *Musculoskeletal health in older women: Impact on fitness, mobility, and functional activity.* Physical Therapy, 91(1), 88-98. https://doi:10.2522/ptj.20100078

Mustard, C. A., Papamichael, C. M., & Brawley, L. R. (2003). *Strength Training in Patients with Type 2 Diabetes: Benefits and Recommendations.* Sports Medicine, 33(2), 117–134. https://doi.org/10.2165/00007256-200333020-00004

Nichols, D. & Sanborn, C.F. (2011). *Bone health in the elderly: Guidelines for identification and management.* American Family Physician, 83(2), 165-173. Retrieved from http://www.aafp.org/afp/2011/0215/p165.html

Noakes, M. (2017). *Exercise, Metabolism and Fitness Over Age 50.* Healthline. https://www.healthline.com/health/exercise-fitness-50

Park, S. T., Lim, S. H., & Do, J. H. (2020). *Effect of resistance exercise on hyperten-*

sion: *A systematic review and meta-analysis*. Sports Medicine, 50(8), 1435–1454. https://doi:10.1007/s40279-020-01271-3

Pointon, M. E., Talbot, D., Anderson, M., & Keogh, J. W. L. (2018). *The Effects of Resistance Training on Glycemic Control Outcomes in Patients with Diabetes Mellitus: A Systematic Review and Meta-Analysis*. Current Diabetes Reports, 18(8), 63. https://doi.org/10.1007/s11892-018-1012-z

PubMed Health. (2007). *Strength Training for Seniors | MedlinePlus*. Retrieved August 25, 2020, from https://medlineplus.gov/strengthtrainingforseniors.html

Rantanen, T., Avila et al. (1998). *Effects of four-month strength-training intervention on muscle strength and physical performance of elderly women*. Age and Ageing, 27(4), 377–384. Retrieved from https://doi.org/10.1093/ageing/27.4.377

Teixeira, V. H., Queiroz, A., Lucinda, J. P., Gomes, C. & Gouveia, M. F. (2017). *Is resistance exercise effective in reducing abdominal visceral fat? A systematic review of randomized controlled trials*. Physiotherapy, 103(2), 118-126. https://doi:10.1016/j.physio.2016.09.002

Thomas, M., Singleton, S., Saxon, L., Tejeda-Burr, A., Ribeiro, O., & White, D. (2018). *Strength Training, Cardiovascular Risk Factors, and Cardiovascular Disease in Adults: A Systematic Review and Meta-Analysis*. Sports Medicine, 48, 321-345.

Truchon, M. S., Bélanger, L., & Llanes, U. J. (2015). *Evidence for physical exercise in the prevention, management and rehabilitation of musculoskeletal disorders among seniors*. Maturitas, 81(2), 237-244. https://doi:10.1016/j.maturitas.2015.04.002

Vieira, V. (2019). *Sarcopenia, Metabolism and Aging: What Is the Link*. Maturitas, 123, 46-50.

Villareal, D., Chode, S., Parimi, N., Sinacore, D., Hilton, T., Armamento-Villareal, R., & Raanes, M. (2017). *Weight Loss, Exercise, or Both and Physical Function in Obese Older Adults*. New England Journal of Medicine, 376, 543-553.

Weatherby, R. P., & Cox, M. H. (2017). *Exercise and cognitive aging*. Clin Geriatr Med, 33(3), 367–376. https://doi:10.1016/j.cger.2017.02.004

Wilson, B. A., Roell, H. A., Dodson, Y., O'Neill-Smithers, M. J., Chou, L. P., & Hutchesson, M. (2020). *Resistance training and cardio exercise: Effects on blood lipids in older adults*. Biology in Sport, 37, 549-558.

World Health Organization. (2018). *Physical activity*. Retrieved 15 October

2020, from https://www.who.int/news-room/fact-sheets/detail/physical-activity

World Health Organization. (2021). *"Cancer Among the Elderly Population"*. Retrieved from https://www.who.int/cancer/prevention/diagnosis-screening/cancer-among-elderly-population

Xing, H. et al. (2017). *The efficacy of strength training for glycemic control in type 2 diabetes patients: A meta-analysis of randomized controlled trials.* Endocrine, 57(2), 343–355. https://doi.org/10.1007/s12020-016-1127-3

Yeh, G. Y., & Haskell, W. L. (2008). *Cardiorespiratory and strength training for older adults: Utilizing American College of Sports Medicine guidelines to gain maximum health benefits.* Clinics in Geriatric Medicine, 25(1), 73-93.

Yeaw, E. et al. (2020). *Exercise-induced muscle damage and its recovery in older adults.* Journal of Physical Therapy Science, 32(11), 1940-1945. https://doi: 10.1589/jpts.32.1940

All images have been sourced from Unsplash.com